Springer Series on Geriatric Nursing

Mathy D. Mezey, RN, EdD, FAAN, Series Editor

2002   **Bathing Without a Battle: Personal Care of Individuals With Dementia**
Ann Louise Barrick, PhD, Joanne Rader, RN, MN, FAAN, Beverly Hoeffer, DNSc, RN, FAAN, and Philip D. Sloane, MD, MPH

2001   **Critical Care Nursing of the Elderly, Second Edition**
Terry T. Fulmer, PhD, RN, FAAN, Marquis D. Foreman, PhD, RN, FAAN, and Mary Walker, PhD, RN, FAAN

1999   **Geriatric Nursing Protocols for Best Practice**
Ivo Abraham, PhD, RN, FAAN, Melissa M. Bottrell, MPH, Terry T. Fulmer, PhD, RN, FAAN, and Mathy D. Mezey, EdD, RN, FAAN

1998   **Home Care for Older Adults: A Guide for Families and Other Caregivers—Text and Instructor's Manual**
Mary Ann Rosswurm, EdD, RN, CS, FAAN

1998   **Restraint-Free Care: Individualized Approaches for Frail Elders**
Neville E. Strumpf, PhD, RN, C, FAAN, Joanne Patterson Robinson, PhD, RN, Joan Stockman Wagner, MSN, CRNP, and Lois K. Evans, DNSc, RN, FAAN

1996   **Gerontology Review Guide for Nurses**
Elizabeth Chapman Shaid, RN, MSN, CRNP, and Kay Huber, DEd, RN, CRNP

1995   **Strengthening Geriatric Nursing Education**
Terry T. Fulmer, RN, PhD, FAAN, and Marianne Matzo, PhD, RN, CS

1994   **Nurse-Physician Collaboration: Care of Adults and the Elderly**
Eugenia L. Siegler, MD, and Fay W. Whitney, PhD, RN, FAAN

1993   **Health Assessment of the Older Individual, Second Edition**
Mathy Doval Mezey, RN, EdD, FAAN, Shirlee Ann Stokes, RN, EdD, FAAN, and Louise Hartnett Rauckhorst, RNC, ANP, EdD

1992   **Critical Care Nursing of the Elderly**
Terry T. Fulmer, RN, PhD, FAAN, and Mary K. Walker, PhD, RN, FAAN

Ann Louise Barrick, PhD is a Clinical Associate Professor at the University of North Carolina at Chapel Hill, Department of Psychology, and Director of Psychology at John Umstead Hospital in Butner, North Carolina. She holds a doctoral degree in Counseling Psychology from Ball State University and has been a geropsychologist since 1986. She provides training to professional staff in the assessment and treatment of persons with dementia. Dr. Barrick has conducted research and published articles addressing behavioral symptoms in dementia, and is coauthor of a training film on methods for bathing persons with dementia.

Joanne Rader, RN, MN, FAAN is an independent consultant and was an Associate Professor at Oregon Health Sciences University School of Nursing. She has worked in the field of long-term care for 30 years. Her work has included funded projects to reduce the use of physical restraints, inappropriate psychoactive medications, and aggressive behaviors during bathing of persons with dementia. She is the author of a 1996 *American Journal of Nursing* Book of the Year entitled *Individualized Dementia Care: Creative, Compassionate Approaches*. Ms. Rader has published numerous articles and books addressing the emotional needs and behavioral symptoms of persons with dementia and recently coauthored and produced manuals and videos on individualized wheelchair seating for older adults. She is a founding member and board member of the Pioneer Network, an organization working to change the culture of aging in America.

Beverly Hoeffer, DNSc, RN, FAAN is a Professor of Nursing and the Associate Dean for Academic Affairs at Oregon Health Sciences University School of Nursing in Portland, Oregon. She received her master's degree in Advanced Psychiatric Nursing from Rutgers University and her doctoral degree in Nursing Science from the University of California, San Francisco. She is a member of the Western Academy of Nurses and a fellow of the American Academy of Nursing. Dr. Hoeffer has conducted research in the area of behavioral symptoms of dementia, including outcome measures and clinical interventions for bathing persons with dementia for the past ten years. She has made numerous presentations and has authored articles and book chapters on the care of persons with dementia.

Philip D. Sloane, MD, MPH is the Elizabeth and Oscar Goodwin Distinguished Professor of Family Medicine at the University of North Carolina at Chapel Hill. A geriatrician, he has served as medical director of several long-term care facilities and has coauthored *Primary Care Geriatrics, Dementia Units in Long-Term Care,* and the Alzheimer's Association's *Key Elements of Dementia Care*. Dr. Sloane is nationally known for his work on the management of persons with Alzheimer's disease and related disorders.

Bathing Without a Battle

Personal Care of Individuals With Dementia

Ann Louise Barrick, *PhD*
Joanne Rader, *MN, RN, FAAN*
Beverly Hoeffer, *DNSc, RN, FAAN*
Philip D. Sloane, *MD, MPH, Editors*

 Springer Publishing Company

Springer Publishing Company, Inc.
536 Broadway
New York, NY 10012-3955

Acquisitions Editor: Ruth Chasek
Production Editor: Sara Yoo
Cover design by Susan Hauley

01 02 03 04 05 / 5 4 3 2 1

Library of Congress Cataloging-in-Publication Data

Bathing without a battle : personal care of individuals with dementia / Ann Louise Barrick . . . [et al.].
   p. cm.
  Includes bibliographical references and index.
  ISBN 0-8261-1507-1
  1. Dementia. 2. Dementia—Patients—Care. 3. Dementia—Patients—Services for. 4. Dementia—Patients—Home care. 5. Baths. 6. Aged—Health and hygiene. I. Barrick, Ann Louise.
  RC521 .B38 2001
  362.1'9683—dc21   2001032246
                                                           CIP

Printed in the United States of America by Capital City Press.

*This book is dedicated to all the direct care workers
who care deeply and struggle daily to provide
compassionate and skillful individualized care.*

Contents

Part III: Supporting Caregiving Activities

Contributors

Cornelia Beck, PhD, RN, FAAN
College of Nursing
University of Arkansas for Medical Services
Little Rock, AR

Margaret P. Calkins, PhD
President
I.D.E.A.S., Inc.
Kirtland, OH

Leanne E. Carnes, BS
Research Assistant
Cecil G. Sheps Center for Health Services Research
University of North Carolina-Chapel Hill
Chapel Hill, NC

Kimberly Horton Hoffman, BS
Infection Control Practitioner
University of Arkansas for Medical Sciences Medical
  Center
Little Rock, AR

Darlene McKenzie, PhD, RN
Professor
School of Nursing
Oregon Health Sciences University
Portland, OR

Debbie Medina
Certified Nursing Assistant
Hood River Care Center
Hood River, OR

Lois L. Miller, PhD, RN
Assistant Professor
School of Nursing
Oregon Health Sciences University
Portland, OR

Madeline Mitchell, MURP
Project Director (NC)
Data Collection/Management
Cecil G. Sheps Center for Health Services Research
University of North Carolina
Chapel Hill, NC

Carla Gene Rapp, PhD, RN, CRRN
Postdoctoral Fellow
Central Arkansas Veterans Health Care System
North Little Rock, AR

Joyce H. Rasin, PhD, RN
Associate Professor
School of Nursing
University of North Carolina
Chapel Hill, NC

Theresa H. Raudsepp, MSPT
Physical Therapist
Providence Benedictine Nursing Center
Mt. Angel, OR

LouAnn Rondorf-Klym, PhD, RN
School of Nursing
Oregon Health Sciences University
Portland, OR

Valorie Shue, BA
Research Assistant
Department of Geriatrics
University of Arkansas for Medical Sciences
Little Rock, AR

Adele Mattinat Spegman, PhD, RN
Senior Research Associate
Oregon Health Sciences University
Portland, OR

Karen Amann Talerico, PhD, RN, CS
Assistant Professor and Scientist
School of Nursing
Oregon Health Sciences University
Portland, OR

Johannah Topps Uriri, MNSc, RNP, CS
College of Nursing
University of Arkansas for Medical Sciences
Little Rock, AR

Jennifer R. Wood, LPTA
Physical Therapy Assistant
Providence Benedictine Nursing Center
Mt. Angel, OR

Preface

The purpose of this book is to change current bathing practices that create unnecessary distress and discomfort for persons with dementia. For many persons, bathing remains a pleasant experience. But, in some cases, bathing becomes a battle for the care recipient and the caregiver. In the last decade we have learned much about ways to improve care for persons with dementia. We have changed many long-held practices and beliefs about what constitutes good care. Yet, many of our standards related to bathing frail elders, particularly those with dementia, remain unchallenged. We hope to change some of your ideas about assisting persons with dementia with bathing by sharing with you lessons we have learned from many years of clinical practice and nine years of conducting research in this area.

THE HISTORY OF OUR APPROACH

The approach to understanding and reducing the distress of bathing persons with dementia presented in this book was developed by two multidisciplinary teams of health care providers and researchers: one at Oregon Health Sciences University (OHSU), the second at the University of North Carolina-Chapel Hill (UNC-CH) and at John Umstead Hospital (JUH), Butner, North Carolina. During the course of our studies we have given over 1000 baths and worked with more than 50 nursing assistants.

We began at UNC-CH and JUH in 1992 with a grant funded by the National Institute of Aging (NIA) as part of a jointly sponsored initiative with the National Institute of Nursing Research (NINR). We found that there were some nursing assistants who seemed to be able to gain the cooperation of patients who were usually aggressive. We watched what they did and talked with them about their approach to care.

From these experiences we learned much about what helps and what makes the bathing experience worse. We had hoped to be able to develop prescriptions for coping with behavioral symptoms such as yelling and hitting, but found that we needed a person-centered, psychosocial, problem-solving approach. This enabled us to tailor each bath to the individual. We tried this approach in two nursing homes and found that we could make most bathing experiences more pleasant. We also found that a bed bath seemed to be more comfortable than a shower or tub bath for the most severely impaired individuals. Having the flexibility to bathe a person in a number of different ways was crucial. However, we knew that we would have to test our ideas in a more rigorous study before we could convince others that a shower or tub bath wasn't the only way to get a person clean.

At the same time the OHSU team was funded by NIA, as part of the same joint initiative with NINR, to conduct a pilot and feasibility study for a clinical trial on changing nursing home staff's approaches to bathing persons with dementia. Our first aim was to gain a better understanding of how much of a problem aggressive behavior was while bathing residents with dementia (e.g., what kinds of behavioral symptoms occurred and how frequently). Our second aim was to determine if a bedside model of consultation between the direct care provider and a clinical nurse specialist, focused on problem solving and individualizing care, would be effective. Both teams found that when we individualized the bath and the bathing care plan we were able to dramatically reduce the aggressive behaviors.

An important insight we gained was that the relationship between the caregiver and care recipient was essential. Nursing assistants who were able to shift from a task-focused to a person-focused approach were more successful in trying new approaches. Another insight was that nursing assistants valued the support they experienced from the consultant for trying new ideas, and expressed that this was often missing from their coworkers or supervisors. Another important "discovery" was that an in-bed towel bath, where the person is fully covered with a towel moistened with no-rinse soap and washed and massaged through the towel, was often comforting and soothing for persons who found even an individualized approach to the shower or tub bath distressing. It was also effective in reducing aggressive behaviors and distress. As a result of the intervention, the nursing assistants who participated also experienced bathing persons with dementia more positively.

Our two teams met because of our mutual interests and decided to join forces in 1995. We believed that our combined approaches from different disciplines (e.g., nursing, medicine, psychology) and the research methods we developed in our first studies would strengthen a larger-scale study across multiple sites. We received funding from the National Institute of Nursing Research to examine two kinds of bathing: shower and in-room bathing in 15 nursing homes in Oregon and North Carolina. Two of the authors (Rader and Barrick) worked side by side with the nursing assistants to learn how to increase pleasure and decrease distress for the residents included in the study.

ABOUT THE BOOK

Out of these experiences we developed our current approach to bathing persons with dementia as discussed in this book. Part I explores bathing from an overall perspective. The model that guides our work is described in Chapter 1. Chapter 2 includes general techniques found to help most persons feel more comfortable during bathing. Chapters 3 and 4 cover assessment and interventions for individualizing bathing plans. They are filled with the many ideas gathered while working with very creative and caring nursing assistants. Part II of the book is devoted to special concerns related to bathing such as pain, skin care, determining the appropriate level of assistance, transfers, and the environment. Part III addresses ways to support caregivers such as training and self-care and also discusses some of the system level issues that can have an impact on caregivers. Several chapters include specific insights and wisdom from direct caregivers.

We worked in health care facilities, but many of the ideas in this book also apply to persons being cared for at home and in other settings such as day care programs. Although we have focused our discussion on persons with dementia, we also believe that many of the approaches discussed in this book are equally useful when caring for other frail elders. Finally, we believe our individualized problem-solving approach and techniques can be useful during other caregiving activities such as morning and evening care.

Our work is not finished. We invite you to use the model and the solutions that we found helpful in your own work. Use your creativity to find the best way to bathe each person in your care. There is no right way to bathe a person, but there are many better ways than current common practices. Bathing can occur without a battle. We hope you will agree.

Acknowledgments

The authors would like to acknowledge the many people who contributed to this book. The research project, Clinical Trial of Two Bathing Interventions in Dementia, on which this book is based, was funded by NINR (R01 NR 04188). We are grateful to NINR for recognizing the importance of this work. The authors thank the members of the interdisciplinary Bathing Project Research Team in Oregon and North Carolina. These include: Darlene A. McKenzie and Joyce H. Rasin (Co-investigators); Barbara Stewart (Psychometrician) and Gary Koch (Biostatistician); C. Madeline Mitchell, Lou-Ann M. Rondorf-Klym, and Adele Mattinat Spegman (Project Directors); Charlene Riedel-Leo, Wilaipun Somboontanont, Karen Amann Talerico, Johannah Uriri, and Virapun Wirojratana (Team Members and Graduate Research Assistants). The authors also thank our consultants: Cornelia Beck, Joyce Colling, Maggie Donius, J. P. Kilborn, and Lynne Morrison. Mary Lavelle contributed generously of her interest, insights and time providing background information about the history of bathing. We also wish to acknowledge the School of Nursing, Oregon Health Sciences University (including Diane Berks, Administrative Assistant), Sheps Center for Health Services Research, University of North Carolina at Chapel Hill and John Umstead Hospital for resources supporting the project.

The following direct caregivers gave generously of their time and efforts to create and share many of the ideas found in the book: Sandra Boedigheimer, Ruth Burt, Laurie Christopherson, Deb Corwin, Edith S. Durham, Kim Francia, Katrina Hardison, Jose Hernandez, Kathy House, Brenda Jantz, Mineko Leavenworth, Debbie Medina, Angell T. Neal, Beth Parker, Lona Pavao, Rosa Sneeds, and Rhonda C. Walton. A special thank you goes to all the facilities, families, residents, and staff who assisted with the project. Without their cooperation and assistance none of this would have been possible.

PART I

The Basics

CHAPTER 1

Understanding the Battle

*Beverly Hoeffer, Joanne Rader,
and Ann Louise Barrick*

Imagine yourself as an older person living in a nursing facility. You grew up at a time when personal care was done in private and seldom discussed. Before you came to the facility, you were used to bathing or showering in a tub in a small warm bathroom that you decorated to your liking many years ago. However, you were having increasing trouble caring for yourself at home because of memory problems, arthritis, and poor balance. After falling and bruising yourself badly, you were admitted to a nursing home following a short hospital stay. Today you are confused and have difficulty remembering where you are or recognizing the people who come into your room. You ache from arthritis in your joints and experience pain when moving your limbs. You are lying in bed, lost in your memories, when suddenly someone tells you it is time for your shower. You can't figure out who this person is, but before you know it, you are swung through the air in a lift and then plunked down on a cold chair that looks like a rolling toilet seat. You cry out because you hurt, but the stranger doesn't seem to notice. She says instead, "This won't take long." Then she strips off your bedclothes, puts a blanket around your shoulders and pulls you backward down the hall in the chair. You feel exposed as cold air hits your bottom and thighs. You are afraid and feel that you have no control over what is happening. Your eyes show your anxiety and you call out, "Help me, help me!" repeatedly, louder and louder. The stranger responds, saying "I'm just taking you to the shower; I'm not going to hurt you," but it doesn't feel that way to you. Then you are in a small room sitting in this toilet seat chair, stripped naked again. The stranger is spraying you with water, asking you, "Is it too hot?" . . . and you cry out, "Too hot, too hot!" And then, "Oh, I'm cold, I'm cold!" She doesn't respond to your cries, but raises your arm up instead. This hurts and you curse her, "Damn you, damn you!" (something you never used to do) and try to push her away. She tells you she is just trying to get the soap off, but you feel assaulted and ignored. You don't want a shower; you don't want someone touching you. You . . . just . . . want . . . out . . . of . . . that . . . room, and away from the spraying water!!

Now, imagine that you are the caregiver trying to help this person take a shower. Bathing is one of the tasks that you are assigned, and you want to do a good job. You like taking care of older people, and the last thing you want to do is cause this person pain or distress. But nothing you say or do seems to help. You steel yourself against her cries and complaints of pain and try to ignore them. Afterward, you are upset with the resident for making you feel so incompetent. You no longer look forward to caring for her because it feels like *such a battle*. You pray that she gets assigned to someone else.

Behavioral Changes in Dementia

The scenario you were asked to imagine describes an all too frequent experience of older persons with dementia and caregivers assigned to help with personal care. With some alterations in the scenario, it could represent the experience of family caregivers when persons with dementia no longer recognize even familiar faces, as can happen in later stages of the illness.

Dementia is not a disease per se, but instead a syndrome characterized by three defining features:

- intellectual deterioration in at least two areas of cognitive functioning (i.e., memory, orientation,

language, judgement, visuospatial skills, concentration, and ability to sequence tasks);
- functional impairment, that is, difficulty carrying out daily activities such as bathing,
- personality changes such as behavioral symptoms (e.g., wandering, physical aggression).

It is accompanied by neuropathology, that is, abnormalities in the central nervous system such as neurofibrillary tangles in Alzheimer's disease (AD) or cerebral infarcts in strokes (Niederehe & Oxman, 1994). The abnormalities in the central nervous system remain invisible to us, revealed only with imaging of the brain through MRIs or CAT scans, and on autopsy.

What the older person with dementia experiences, and what we as caregivers observe, are the changes in behavior and ways of communicating caused by brain disease. From the caregiver's perspective, these behavioral symptoms are often viewed as "defiant behaviors," "problematic" or "troublesome" behavior, or "disruptive behaviors." Often this perspective implies that the person with dementia is the problem or is having a problem that needs to be managed. If we turn the lens around and look at behavioral symptoms from the view of the person receiving care, a much different perspective emerges. Behavioral symptoms become ways of communicating experiences such as:

- fear, pain or distress
- expressions of unmet or unidentified needs
- self-protective behavior against an invasion of personal space or feeling assaulted.

Ultimately, behavior becomes the primary means of communicating for persons with dementia when they are no longer able to express their feelings, needs, or desires verbally, or to engage in problem solving with others.

As the population ages, dementia is becoming an increasingly significant health problem that is likely to touch all of our lives in some way. Alzheimer's disease (AD) is the most common cause of dementia among older persons, affecting approximately four million persons or 10.9% of the older population (National Institute on Aging, 1999). The prevalence of AD increases with age and, in fact, doubles every five years beyond age 65 (Administration on Aging, 1999). A large community-based study found that just 3% of persons 65–74 years and 18.7% of persons 75–84 years had AD; however,

nearly half (47%) of persons 85 and older had AD (Evans et al., 1989). The majority of persons with AD are cared for at home, although many families turn to facilities to provide the 24-hour care required in the later stages of this progressive illness. Declining abilities to carry out activities of daily living (ADLs) and increasing occurrences of behavioral symptoms during assistance with personal care are often factors that lead to nursing home placement.

Prevalence of Behavioral Symptoms During Bathing

We know that behavioral symptoms of dementia that occur when assisting persons with personal care activities such as bathing are among the most troublesome and difficult for caregivers. Within community settings, family members surveyed in one study reported that 65% of persons with dementia they cared for had become aggressive during caregiving (Ryden, 1988). In another study, family members reported increases in the number of persons with behavioral symptoms as cognitive impairment became more severe (Teri, Larson, & Reifer, 1988). They also indicated that assisting with hygiene precipitated the most problematic behaviors. Within nursing homes, behavioral symptoms ranged from an average prevalence of 43% among all persons across a number of studies (Beck, Rossby, & Baldwin, 1991; Beck et al., 1998) to 86% of persons with dementia (Ryden, Bossenmaier, & McLachlan, 1991). In the latter study, nearly three-quarters (72.3%) of aggressive behavior among 124 nursing home residents occurred during caregiving activities involving touch or invasion of personal space.

When caregivers are asked about behavioral symptoms that occur during assistance with personal care such as bathing, they describe behaviors that fall into three general categories. These include:

- resistive behaviors (e.g., pulls away to avoid being bathed; tries to leave bathing area)
- vocal agitation or distress (e.g., crying, loud exclamations such as Oh! Oh!)
- verbal and physical aggression (e.g., cursing, threatening, hitting, biting, grabbing, pushing).

To better describe behavioral symptoms that occur during bathing and the extent to which bathing persons with dementia is difficult for caregivers in nursing facilities, study teams in Oregon and North Carolina conducted two surveys. In Oregon, the team collected in-depth data on all residents in one nursing home over a 6-week period (Hoeffer, Rader, McKenzie, Lavelle, & Stewart, 1997). Most residents were bathed weekly in this facility. At the beginning of the survey, 93 of the 102 long-stay residents (91%) required assistance with bathing. Eighty-six of these residents remained in the facility throughout the 6-week period and were included in the study. The nursing assistants who helped residents with bathing completed a checklist of physical, verbal, and sexually aggressive behaviors. The team analyzed data from the first four baths for each resident. Nearly half (41%) were aggressive during at least one of the four baths, and a significant number (16%) were aggressive almost every time (i.e., during three of the four baths). The majority of residents (60%) who were aggressive during one bath had a diagnosis of dementia, and an even higher percent (72%) who were aggressive during almost every bath had a dementia diagnosis. Of those residents who were aggressive during bathing, 63% were both physically and verbally aggressive. Very few residents were sexually aggressive during bathing. By far the most frequent types of physically aggressive behaviors reported by nursing assistants in descending order of frequency were:

- hitting, punching or slapping
- pinching or squeezing
- pushing or shoving.

Verbally aggressive behaviors reported were fairly evenly distributed among:

- the use of hostile language
- name-calling
- cursing or obscene language.

Aggressive behavior occurred most frequently during the bath itself, but also during undressing and transportation to the bath. The nursing assistants reported other kinds of behaviors not included on the checklist that they found troublesome. These included vocal agitation such as:

- crying
- calling out
- yelling.

The bathing study team in North Carolina team took a different approach to learning more about the extent of the problem. They conducted a survey of 60 nursing homes in North Carolina, drawn randomly from a list of licensed facilities in the state, and of 54 facilities nationwide operated by one proprietary group (Sloane et al., 1995). A questionnaire was mailed to the director of nursing or charge nurse familiar with bathing-related issues in each facility. The response rate was 62%, lending credibility to the results. Half of the 71 facilities that completed the survey had special care units for persons with Alzheimer's disease.

Over three-quarters of residents usually received a shower which was almost always given in a common bathing area. Very few received a bed bath in their own room. Only half of the nurses reported that they were satisfied with the bathing process in their facility. On average 20% of the residents were reported to be difficult to bathe. Of the residents who were reported as difficult to bathe, 81% had a diagnosis of dementia. The kinds of behaviors reported as common among residents with dementia who were difficult to bathe were similar to those reported by the caregivers in the Oregon survey. Behaviors reported at least half of the time included physically and verbally aggressive behaviors, resistive behaviors, and vocal agitation.

We know less about the prevalence of behavioral symptoms when family members assist persons with dementia during bathing. One study of 64 family caregivers of persons with dementia found that 41% assisted their family member during bathing; of these about half found doing so "pretty hard" or "somewhat hard" (Archbold et al., 1997).

When Does the Battle Begin?

We often think of bathing as the time that a person spends in the bath or shower. But in caregiving situations, bathing begins with the invitation to the bath. The invitation to the bath is a pivotal time for the battle to start or be prevented. Bathing-related activities during which the battle can occur or be prevented include:

- undressing and dressing
- transfer between the bed or bathtub and a chair
- transportation to the bath or shower room
- the bath or shower procedures, including washing and drying
- hair washing or shaving.

It is not the activity itself that causes the behavioral symptoms but rather the person's experience of the situation from the time of the invitation to the completion of the bath. The most frequent antecedents or causes of behavioral symptoms during personal care activities such as bathing reported in the literature include:

- touch or invasion of personal space
- perceived loss of control or choice
- anticipation or experience of pain
- feeling that one's needs and preferences are being ignored
- frustration experienced because of declining self-care abilities
- impaired ability to express or communicate needs or feelings
- impaired ability to recognize caregiver's actions as helpful
- tense caregiver appearance, nonengaged communication, or tasked-oriented behavior.

Because persons with dementia may no longer be able to recognize the caregiver's actions as helpful, they may feel threatened by the invitation to the bath and perceive the bath as an assault. Resistive and aggressive behaviors are, in essence, a defensive response to a perceived threat (Bridges-Parlet, Knopman, & Thompson, 1994), a way for persons to "fight back" in an attempt to prevent harm from occurring to them during bathing.

A useful way to think about the battle is to view it as a conflict between the agendas of the caregiver and the person with dementia. In an observational study of 33 persons with dementia during bath time, Kovach and Meyer-Arnold (1996; 1997) found that 92% became agitated or resistive as soon as they were told that it was time to take a bath. The high prevalence of behavioral symptoms during the invitation to the bath suggests *conflicting agendas* between the person with dementia and the caregiver *from the beginning*. The caregiver feels that he or she must give the bath, and the person with dementia, who does not want the bath, feels little control over the situation. Both cope with their conflicting agendas through verbal and nonverbal strategies, all of which have meaning within the context of the bathing situation. Persons with dementia cope with their loss of control through behaviors that reflect attempts at sharing control, resigning control, attaining control, and/or regaining inner control. Behavioral symptoms,

including resistive behaviors, vocal agitation, and physical and verbal aggression, occur most often during attempts to attain control or to regain inner control.

Kovach and Meyer-Arnold (1996, 1997) also found that specific communication styles and actions of caregivers were related to the occurrence of either calm behavior or agitated behavior by the persons being bathed. Engaged communication included:

- conversation about general topics with the person
- attention to the person's need for comfort and personal preferences during bathing
- reassuring, explaining, and comforting phrases
- diversion
- requests for the person's participation
- humor and compliments.

Nonengaged communications included:

- talking to another caregiver rather than the person
- firm directives and coaxing
- degrading comments and jokes at the person's expense.

A person-focused approach, paced to meet the needs of the person being bathed, rather than a task-oriented approach, often rushed to meet the needs of the caregiver, is the key to preventing the battle from the beginning. It serves to calm the person and help him or her to cope more successfully with the situation.

The physical environment can also contribute to behavioral symptoms during bathing. Environmental factors leading to discomfort and apprehension, often expressed as resistive, agitated, or aggressive behavioral symptoms include:

- unfamiliar appearance of bathing rooms in facilities
- bathing apparatus and transportation equipment
- the temperature of the room and the water
- spraying and running water
- loud or unusual noises.

Consequently, the battle can be precipitated by events in the physical environment that affect the experience of persons with dementia and caregivers.

Moreover, caregivers report that the support they perceive from their coworkers and supervisors, and from the culture in the facility, influences how they approach bathing persons with dementia. Factors that affect this "caregiving tone" include:

- philosophy
- policy and procedures
- staffing patterns
- structure of day
- equipment and supplies.

The importance of these organizational factors on interactive caregiving is critical. They control how much flexibility, personability, and caregiving creativity the organization will accept and support. Sometimes caregivers are pressured to conform to rigid policies, procedures and schedules. Other times, the open, facilitative tone set by the administration gets lost or distorted as it travels to those directly interacting with people with dementia.

Some facilities allow only one towel and one washcloth per bath. This makes it difficult to keep the person covered and warm. Other facilities require showers and do not allow bed baths. In homes, there may be rigid beliefs about how to help someone stay clean or when baths can or can't be done. Such policies and beliefs can set the stage for a battle.

Thus, interventions aimed at making bath time a more positive and pleasant experience must take into account the organizational and physical environments that help shape the psychosocial or interpersonal environment in which bathing occurs.

Addressing Myths About Bathing

There are some strongly held beliefs about what is required to keep people clean that need to be addressed. Most of us resist change. It is generally "easier" to do what we have always done. To champion change related to bathing, a number of myths about bathing have to be confronted and overcome. Some common ones to consider are:

- **You have to use lots of water to get clean.**

    Many conscientious caregivers worry that they need to use lots of water in the shower, bath, or bed. However, people have maintained cleanliness without the benefit of showers, tubs, or running water at home and in other settings. Careful washing with attention to detail is more important than how much water you use.

- **If caregivers are delaying, deferring, shortening, or adapting the bath or shower, they are trying to get out of work.**

    This is not about being lazy. It may be necessary to create an individualized plan that meets the person's special needs. Caregivers are still responsible for maintaining the person's hygiene but need freedom to adjust the method. Altering the bathing method or schedule actually may reflect the caregiver's commitment to good care and being conscientious rather that trying to get out of work.

- **Families will insist on a shower or tub bath.**

    Families, like the rest of us, need to be educated. If they are presented with the problem (e.g., the person dislikes or fights the bath or shower) and alternative suggestions, families usually understand and are agreeable to trying other methods.

- **There will be more infections and skin problems.**

    In our culture, especially during the twentieth century, we have associated the importance of bathing with preventing health problems. However, our experience suggests that modifying the bathing experience and using methods other than the routine bath or shower and plenty of regular soap does not result in more skin problems or infections. The use of an alternative no-rinse soap solution may prevent some skin problems such as drying and allergic reactions to soap products.

- **People always feel better after they have a bath or shower and are clean.**

    Just because we feel better after a bath or shower does not mean others do, particularly when it is uncomfortable or they clearly state they don't want it and it is forced upon them. In these cases the person feels distressed or violated.

- **You have to just go ahead because for most people who resist, there won't be a "good" time.**

For most people with dementia, developing a plan that keeps them clean and avoids the battle *is* possible. When the approach, method, day, and time of day are adjusted to the person's needs, bathing without a battle is almost always the outcome.

- **They just forget about the battle so it doesn't matter.**

  Many people who are forced to bathe stay upset for hours following the task. It is almost as if our care plans say, "agitate to the point of aggression one to two times a week during bathing." If the person feels he/she is being forced or threatened on a regular basis during bathing, our experience suggests that even with memory loss there can be a lasting effect on his/her overall feelings of safety and well-being. Examples of lasting outcomes from forced bathing could include refusal to take medicines, aggressive confrontations with other residents, or further resistance with staff in other care areas.

- **Regulators, advocates, and families will see it as possible neglect.**

  When you are changing what is currently accepted practice, proactively educating all players, particularly those who may be most critical, is an important strategy. As was the case with changing practice related to restraints, the risk of being misjudged is greater if the only message given is what is not being done, rather than the more positive message about the efforts being made towards individualizing care. The goal is to provide good care by meeting the unique needs of persons with dementia and avoiding distressing bathing situations. Plans for evaluating problems and monitoring improvement also need to be presented.

- **An individualized approach will take more time, and we don't have time for extra care.**

  For most persons, individualized care can be done in the same amount of time as routine care once you are familiar with the new methods, approaches, and techniques. If you end up bathing some people less frequently, then there may be a decrease in overall time spent bathing.

The Impact of the Battle

What happens if the battle is not prevented or mitigated in some way? What are the consequences for persons with dementia and caregivers? If you have experienced the battle yourself or observed its occurrence at home or in a nursing facility, then the consequences may sound all too familiar. Besides experiencing the battle during the bathing situation, persons with dementia may remain upset and agitated the remainder of the day, affecting their relationships with others with whom they have daily contact. The result is that they may be avoided by others and become increasingly isolated and depressed. Often they become perceived as difficult and troublesome. Too often the outcome has been the misuse of psychoactive medications to control behavioral symptoms or the use of physical restraints (Talerico, Evans, & Strumpf, 2000). We usually think of physical restraints as tying someone down, but other forms of restraint include using three to four caregivers to hold a person against his/her will while the bath is given quickly.

Behavioral symptoms, especially aggressive behavior, have serious consequences for caregivers in community and nursing home settings. Caregivers in nursing facilities have rated assisting persons with dementia during bathing or showering as one of the hardest, if not the most difficult, caregiving task that they perform (Namazi, 1996; Miller, 1997). Caregivers experience distress and frustration with the caregiving role, and may become depressed about their situation. Ultimately, this leads to caregiver burnout and a sense that the burden of caregiving is too great. For family caregivers, the result may be that they are no longer able to provide the care at home. In nursing facilities, the result is often low staff morale and high staff turnover. A recent study (Miller, 1997), in which in-depth interviews were conducted with 30 nursing staff in a Dementia Special Care Unit, examined the effects of physically aggressive behavior during hygienic care on staff personally and on their practice. Personally, staff reported declines in their physical health, such as pain and exhaustion, and in their mental health. Mental health status declines included:

- worry about their safety during caregiving
- mental exhaustion, frustration, anger, sadness, depression, and anxiety

- fear of being perceived as a poor worker by their peers or administration.

Their daily experiences with aggressive behavior during caregiving also resulted in changes in their practice, including:

- decline in the perceived quality of nursing care given
- increase in the potential for staff-to-patient abuse and neglect
- desire to eventually leave the unit, the facility, or the profession.

The findings for this qualitative in-depth study confirm the results from surveys and anecdotal reports of caregivers' experiences in the literature.

Conclusions

The costs of the battle are high: for persons with dementia who no longer feel in control of their lives and are avoided by others; for caregivers who feel burdened and distressed by the experience; and for facilities faced with constant turnover. The answer lies in challenging the myths and changing the experience for all involved by finding new ways that bathing can occur without a battle.

REFERENCES

Archbold, P., Kaye, J., Keane, T., Lear, J., Miller, F., Parker, N., & Stewart, B. J. (1997). Family caregiving inventory: The caregiver's perspective. Unpublished data.

Administration on Aging (1999). Alzheimer's disease: Aging fact sheet. [Online] www.aoa.dhhs.gov/factsheets/alz.html (retrieved February, 2000).

Beck, C., Frank, L., Chumbler, N., O'Sullivan, P., Vogelpohl, T., Rasin, J., Walls, R., & Baldwin, B. (1998). Correlates of disruptive behavior in severely cognitively impaired nursing home residents. *The Gerontologist, 38*(2), 189–198.

Beck, C., Rossby, L., & Baldwin, B. (1991). Correlates of disruptive behavior in cognitively impaired elderly nursing home residents. *Archives of Psychiatric Nursing, 5*(5), 281–291.

Bridges-Parlet, S., Knopman, D., & Thompson, T. (1994). A descriptive study of physically aggressive behavior in dementia by direct observation. *Journal of the American Geriatrics Society, 42*(2), 192–197.

Burgener, S. C., Jirovec, M., Murrell, L., & Barton, D. (1992). Caregiver and environmental variables related to difficult behaviors in institutionalized, demented elderly persons. *Journal of Gerontology, 47*(4), 242–249.

Chrisman, M., Tabar, D., Whall, A. L., & Booth, D. E. (1991). Agitated behavior in the cognitively impaired elderly. *Journal of Gerontological Nursing, 17*(12), 9–13.

Cohen-Mansfield, J., Marx, M. S., & Rosenthal, A. S. (1990). Dementia and agitation in nursing home residents: How are they related? *Psychology & Aging, 5*(1), 3–8.

Cohen-Mansfield, J., Marx, M. S., & Werner, P. (1992). Agitation in elderly persons: An integrative report of findings in a nursing home. *International Psychogeriatrics, 4*(Suppl. 2), 221–240.

Evans, D., Funkenstein, H., Albert, M., Scherr, P., Cook, N., Chown, M., Hebert, L., Hennekens, C., & Taylor, J. (1989). Prevalence of Alzheimer's disease in a community population of older persons. *Journal of the American Medical Association, 262*, 2551–2556.

Feldt, K. S., Warne, M. A., & Ryden, M. B. (1998). Examining pain in aggressive cognitively impaired older adults. *Journal of Gerontological Nursing, 24*(11), 14–22.

Hoeffer, B., Rader, J., McKenzie, D., Lavelle, M., & Stewart, B. (1997). Reducing aggressive behavior during bathing cognitively impaired nursing home residents. *Journal of Gerontological Nursing, 23*(5), 16–23.

Jackson, M. E., Drugovich, M. L., Fretwell, M. D., Spector, W. D., Sternberg, J., & Rosenstein, R. B. (1989). Prevalence and correlates of disruptive behavior in the nursing home. *Journal of Aging and Health, 1*(3), 349–369.

Kolanowski, A., Garr, M., Evans, L. K., & Strumpf, N. E. (1998). Behavioral syndromes in institutionalized elders. *American Journal of Alzheimer's Disease, Sept (Oct)*, 245–256.

Kovach, C. R., & Meyer-Arnold, E.A. (1996). Coping with conflicting agendas: The bathing experience of cognitively impaired older adults. *Scholarly Inquiry for Nursing Practice: An International Journal, 10*(1), 23–36.

Kovach, C. R., & Meyer-Arnold, E. A. (1997). Preventing agitated behaviors during bath time. *Geriatric Nursing, 18*(3), 112–114.

Malone, M. L., Thompson, L., & Goodwin, J. S. (1993). Aggressive behaviors among the institutionalized elderly. *Journal of the American Geriatric Society, 41*(8), 853–856.

Marx, M. S., Werner, P., & Cohen-Mansfield, J. (1989). Agitation and touch in the nursing home. *Psychological Reports, 64*(3 Pt. 2), 1019–1026.

Maxfield, M. C., Lewis, R. E., & Cannon, S. (1996). Training staff to prevent aggressive behavior of cognitively impaired elderly patients during bathing and grooming. *Journal of Gerontological Nursing, 22*(1), 37–43.

McShane, R. E. (1996). Response to "Coping with conflicting agendas: The bathing experience of cognitively impaired older adults". *Scholarly Inquiry for Nursing Practice, 10*(1), 37–42.

Meddaugh, D. I. (1990). Reactance: Understanding aggressive behavior in long-term care. *Journal of Psychosocial Nursing & Mental Health Services, 28*(4), 28–33.

Miller, M. F. (1997). Physically aggressive behavior during hygienic care. *Journal of Gerontological Nursing, 23*(5), 24–39.

Miller, R. I. (1994). Managing disruptive responses to bathing by elderly residents: Strategies for the cognitively impaired. *Journal of Gerontological Nursing, 20*(11), 35–39.

National Institute on Aging. (1999). Progress Report on Alzheimer's Disease (NIH Publication No. 99-4664). Washington, DC: U.S. Government Printing Office.

Namazi, K. H., & Johnson, B. D. (1996). Issues related to behavior and the physical environment: Bathing cognitively impaired patients. *Geriatric Nursing, 17*(5), 234–238; quiz 238–239.

Niederehe, G., & Oxman, T. E. (1994). The dementias: Construct and nosologic validity. In V. O. Emery & T. E. Oxman (Eds.), *Dementia: Presentations, differential diagnosis, and nosology* (pp. 19–45). Baltimore, MD: The Johns Hopkins University Press.

Rader, J. (1994). To bathe or not to bathe: That is the question. *Journal of Gerontological Nursing, 20*(9), 53–54.

Rader, J., Lavelle, M., Hoeffer, B., & McKenzie, D. (1996). Maintaining cleanliness: An individualized approach. *Journal of Gerontological Nursing, 22*(3), 32–38.

Rossby, L., Beck, C., & Heacock, P. (1992). Disruptive behaviors of a cognitively impaired nursing home resident. *Archives of Psychiatric Nursing, 6*(2), 98–107.

Ryden, M. B. (1988). Aggressive behavior in persons with dementia who live in the community. *Alzheimer's Disease and Associated Disorders, 2*(4), 342–355.

Ryden, M. B., Bossenmaier, M., & McLachlan, C. (1991). Aggressive behavior in cognitively impaired nursing home residents. *Research in Nursing & Health, 14*(2), 87–95.

Sloane, P. D., Honn, V. J., Dwyer, S. A., Wieselquist, J., Cain, C., & Myers, S. (1995a). Bathing the Alzheimer's patient in long-term care: Results and recommendations from three studies. *American Journal of Alzheimer's Care and Related Disorders & Research,* July/August, 3–11.

Sloane, P. D., Rader, J., Barrick, A., Hoeffer, B., Dwyer, S., McKenzie, D., Lavelle, M., Buckwalter, K., Arrington, L., & Pruitt, T. (1995b). Bathing persons with dementia. *Gerontologist, 35*(5), 672–678.

Talerico, K., Evans, L., & Strumpf, N. (2000). Mental health correlates of aggressive behavior in dementia. (Manuscript submitted for publication).

Teri, L., Larson, E. B., & Reifer, B. V. (1988). Behavioral disturbance in dementia of the Alzheimer's type. *Journal of the American Geriatrics Society, 36*(1), 1–6.

Winger, J., Schirm, V., & Stewart, D. (1987). Aggressive behavior in long-term care. *Journal of Psychosocial Nursing & Mental Health Services, 25*(4), 28–33.

CHAPTER 2

General Guidelines for Bathing Persons With Dementia

Ann Louise Barrick, Joanne Rader, and Debbie Medina

GUIDELINES FOR BATHING WITHOUT A BATTLE

Bathing is a particularly sensitive issue for persons with dementia. People with brain disease become confused easily and often misinterpret what others are doing or saying. In such individuals, often even the smallest thing that is unpleasant such as water in the eyes or ears can make them respond with fear or violence. These responses are not something the person can control. Keep these general guidelines in mind when bathing every person:

- *Focus more on the person than the task.* Meeting individual preferences and emphasizing the well-being of the person being bathed is more important than providing care in an efficient manner. The "car-wash approach" may get the person clean but the cost to both you and the other person is high. Observe the person's feelings and reactions. (Is there fear/pain?) Always protect privacy and dignity.
- *Be flexible.* Modify your approach to meet the needs of the person. This involves adapting: 1) your methods (e.g., distracting the person with singing while bathing); 2) the physical environment (e.g., choosing correct size of shower chair); and 3) the procedure (e.g., dividing up tasks such as hair washing and bathing).
- *Use persuasion, not coercion.* Help the person feel in control. Give choices and respond to individual requests. Support remaining abilities. Negotiate or find a reason that the person can accept. The goal is for you to help the person to get to "yes." Use shortcuts such as no-rinse soap.

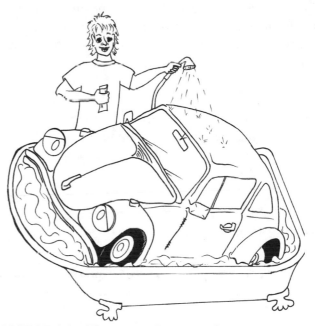

FIGURE 2.1   The car-wash approach.

Use distractions such as food or conversation when necessary to help the person feel more pleasure. Use a supportive, calm approach and praise the person often.
- *Be prepared.* Gather everything you will need for the bath before approaching the person. Where will the bath take place? In the person's room? In the bathroom? Warm the room. What special products will you need? Do you have enough towels? Washcloths? If the person likes to be dressed in the bathroom, do you have all of the person's clothes?
- *Stop.* When a person becomes distressed, stop and assess the situation. It is not "normal" for a

11

person to cry, moan, or fight during bathing. Look for the underlying reason for the behavior. What can you do to prevent the person from becoming more upset?

- *Ask for help.* Talking with others about ways to meet the needs of the person gives you an opportunity to find different ways to help make the bath more comfortable.

GENERAL STRATEGIES FOR STOPPING THE BATTLE

Simple interventions can often be surprisingly effective in reducing the stress of the bathing experience for you and the person you are bathing. These can be divided into five areas:

- meeting personal needs
- adapting interpersonal/relationship factors
- adapting the physical environment
- adapting the organizational environment
- stopping the battle.

Meeting Personal Needs

The most common personal needs expressed by elders during bathing are freedom from pain, cold, and fear, and a wish for a sense of control over what happens to them. Strategies for addressing the needs of most elderly people include these:

- Cover! Cover! Cover! Keep the person covered as much as possible or desired to keep them warm and minimize muscle tension. Wash one area at a time and then cover the area.
- Time the bath to fit the person's history, preferences, and mood.
- Bathe the person before she or he is dressed for the day to eliminate extra movement and discomfort.
- Move slowly and prepare the person prior to moving him/her by counting or giving a warning.
- Watch out for legs and other body parts that might get bumped or injured when moving.
- Minimize the number of moves during the bath.

- Evaluate the need for medical treatments for pain control.
- Start with the least sensitive area so that pain and tension do not immediately escalate. Wash the most sensitive area (as defined by the person being bathed) last.
- Ask the person who is able to talk what will help him or her feel better.
- Use soft cloths such as baby washcloths on sensitive skin.
- Use a gentle touch.
- Pat dry rather than rub to decrease discomfort.
- If the person is fearful of tubs with mechanical lifts, use another method for bathing.

Adapting Interpersonal/Relationship Factors

The relationship between you and the person you are bathing is enhanced by the following general approaches:

- Address the person by his/her preferred name.
- Encourage self-care if appropriate.
- Engage the person in conversation (talk about things, events, and persons of interest to the person; ask the person's opinion).
- Give compliments and praise.
- Tell the person what you are doing at all times and avoid surprises.

Caregiver Wisdom

You have to try to get the person to trust you. The relationship is really important. Sit and talk with the person. Know what their needs are. If you tell someone you are going to do something, always do it. Everyone needs a friendly face and a kind word.
    Ruth Burt, CNA, Oxford Manor, Oxford, NC

- Adjust your language to match the person's ability to understand (see chapter 8). Use verbal interventions with persons who can still talk, and pay special attention to nonverbal behaviors with persons who cannot talk.
- Follow the person's lead. Talk if the person responds and is not overwhelmed. Sing if the person

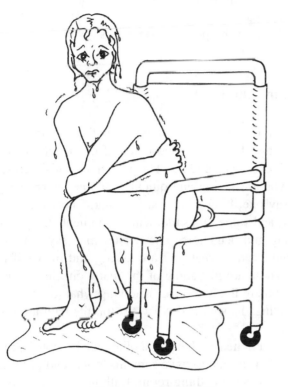

Person wet and cold.

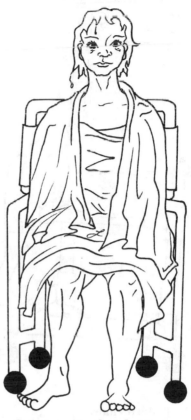

Person covered and warm.

FIGURE 2.2   Covering can make a big difference.

likes it. Be silent if that works best. Too much talking can increase agitation in some people.

- Avoid the word "bath" with persons who do not like to bathe. Use an expression that is acceptable (e.g., wash up).
- Speak calmly, slowly, and simply while facing the person.
- Apologize repeatedly at any sign of distress.
- Go slow, giving the person enough time to process your questions and requests.
- Provide gentle, reassuring touch, if tolerated and desired.
- Use distractions such as objects to hold, candy, or other food that the person likes, to help soothe the person and give him something else to do. Use caution in offering food. Check for dietary and swallowing restrictions first.
- Let the person know what is left to do (e.g., "I'll wash your back and then we are done").

Adapting the Physical Environment

The temperature of the bathing room, the design and comfort of the shower chair, lighting, noise, and sense of privacy all affect the person's experience of bathing. Try the following suggestions to modify the physical environment and make the bath more pleasant:

- Pad the shower chair to increase comfort (Figure 2.3). Padded shower chairs can be purchased. However, if this is not an option, use of a padded child's toilet seat insert, or washcloths around the edge of the seat can also increase comfort.
- Turn the heat on or run the hot water in the bathroom prior to giving a bath and give the room time to warm up.
- Adapt the equipment so it fits the person. For example, for a small person, use a short shower chair or a stool with a standard chair to keep the

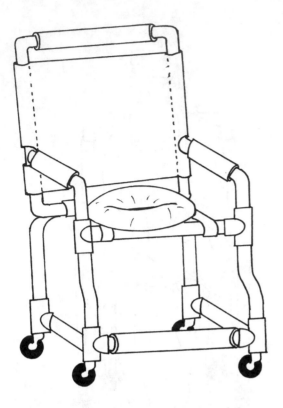

FIGURE 2.3   Padded chair.

feet from dangling and to promote a feeling of security and safety.

- Use beds that can be raised or lowered as needed for staff and resident safety and comfort.
- Reduce noise levels and/or provide soothing music.

Adapting the Organizational Environment

Rigid policies and practices related to acceptable frequency and types of bathing will hamper your ability to provide individualized care. Some possible ways to modify the organizational environment include:

- Use consistent assignment of caregivers so there is an opportunity to get to know the person and establish a relationship.
- Encourage flexibility in schedules for baths. If a person prefers a bath in the evening, arrange to have it done then.
- Use two care providers if needed.

- Try a bed bath if a tub bath or shower causes distress.
- Invite family members to give input or help with the bath.
- Respect the person's right to say "no."

Stopping the Bath

When you are caring for someone with dementia, it is frustrating when your kindest, best efforts result in your being kicked and yelled at. The person may misinterpret what you are saying and quickly become angry. They may say one thing and mean another. There are day-to-day, and some times moment-to-moment changes in thinking and behaviors. The person may say that he/she understands what you are asking and then fail to do it. These are just some of the many puzzling situations you are likely to face. Knowing what to do when these things happen and when to stop the bath are important.

As mentioned earlier, it should not be considered standard or normal to have screams, cries, and protests coming from the bathing room. Bathing battles are potentially harmful physically and emotionally to both parties. When signs of distress occur during a bath follow these steps:

1. Stop what you are doing.
2. Assess for causes of distress.
3. Adjust your approach.
4. Evaluate the effectiveness of the new approach.
5. Shorten or stop the bath.
6. Try to end on a positive note before you leave.
7. Reapproach later to finish washing critical areas if necessary.

If you are unable to calm the person and make the bath more comfortable, you will need to shorten the bath. If the person is very aggressive, you will need to stop the bath. Wash only what is necessary for good health. If the person becomes so distressed you must end the bath, try to end with something pleasant, such as offering a cup of coffee or a back rub. This may make it easier when you return. The next two chapters contain ideas to use when these general strategies do not reduce the stress of the bath.

NOTE

The material in this chapter was adapted with permission from: Rader, J., & Barrick, A. L. (2000). Ways that work: Bathing without a battle, *Alzheimer's Care Quarterly, 1*(4), 35–49.

CHAPTER 3

Assessing Behaviors

*Ann Louise Barrick, Joanne Rader,
and Madeline Mitchell*

The general strategies in chapter 2 can help bathing be more pleasant. To get the best results, especially in difficult cases, you need to tailor your care to the specific needs of the person. This requires knowing a lot about the person, having a large number of options handy, and being flexible. The next two chapters prepare you for this individualized, person-centered approach. This is a continuous process that is useful anytime there is evidence of distress. The steps include:

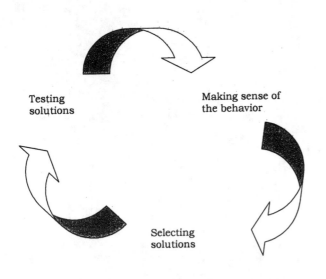

Testing solutions

Making sense of the behavior

Selecting solutions

MAKING SENSE OF THE BEHAVIOR

Being nice is not enough! We observed many caregivers using a calm, gentle approach. But without understanding why the person is resisting or distressed, they were unable to make a difference. Understanding the meaning of behavioral symptoms, from the person's perspective, and seeing them as an expression of a problem or need

will open up a wide range of solutions. This requires a careful assessment of the person and the behavior to uncover the trigger(s) or cause(s) of the behavior.

Understand the Person

Knowing as much as you can about the person will help you understand why the behavior might be occurring as well as choose strategies to reduce it. The Personal Information Data Sheet (see chapter appendix) can be used for gathering the following information:

- **Personal history:** What are the person's past accomplishments, topics of interest, family relations, hobbies, likes and dislikes?
- **Physical health:** Find out the person's remaining abilities as well as problems including mobility, areas of pain, sensitivity to cold, medications, visual and hearing impairments, and diseases. Knowledge of current health problems that may cause behaviors is crucial.
- **Personality factors:** Does the person have a sense of humor? Is he/she outgoing and gregarious or introverted and quiet? Has a need for control been important?
- **Psychosocial well-being and mood:** Is the person involved and interested in daily activities? Is there any evidence of depression? Are there friends and family that visit?
- **Preferences for bathing:** Find out about past bathing habits as well as the current preferred time of day and type of bath. The Bathing Preferences and Practices Form (see chapter appendix) can be given to the family to gather this information.

- **Level of dementia:** How does the person communicate? Are there memory impairments, difficulty with attention, impaired judgment, or impulse control?

Sources of this information include:

- the person
- the family
- other caregivers
- other staff (housekeepers, dietary, social services, activities)
- medical/clinical record.

Caregiver Wisdom

Start by getting to know each other. Tell them who you are and what you are there to do. Learn as much as you can about them. Make sure that you are talking to them at eye level and that they can hear you. You need to have at least a bit of a relationship before you start having them undress. They need to have a sense that you are there to help and not to hurt them.

Debbie Medina, CNA, Hood River
Care Center, Hood River, OR

Describe the Behavior

Work on only one behavior at a time. Although there may be several different behaviors causing concern, choose the one that is most upsetting, such as hitting. Observe the person carefully when the behavior occurs. Gather as much information as you can about this behavior. The Behavior Tracking Log (Figure 3.1) can be used to document your observations and answers to the following questions about the behavior:

- What is the person doing that indicates that the person is distressed (e.g., crying, yelling, grabbing, trying to hit, trying to leave)?
- When does the behavior occur (e.g., when the water is turned on, during cleansing of the feet)?
- Is this a new behavior?
- Where does the behavior occur (e.g., in the shower room but not the bedroom)?
- Who is involved when this happens?

- How often does this happen?
- What happens just before the behavior?
- What happens after?
- What seems to help?
- What seems to make the behavior worse?
- What makes this behavior a concern?

These questions help you identify **behavioral triggers.** Triggers may be people, places, or events that cause the behavior to occur or get worse. Sometimes behaviors have multiple triggers. Refusing to enter the shower room may be triggered by modesty, physical discomfort of a shower chair, or fear of being cold.

Look for Causes/Triggers of the Behavior

Every behavior has meaning but often the meaning has to be uncovered or discovered. This may be a difficult process as behaviors are complex and may have many different triggers. You have to figure out what the person is trying to communicate. Try viewing the bath through the eyes, ears, and feelings of the person. For example, think about:

- How do you respond if you think a stranger is trying to take your clothes off?
- How does it feel to have water that is too hot or too cold hitting you?
- What might help to make you more comfortable?

Look for the cause of the behaviors anytime there is a sign of discomfort. Systematic observation is crucial. Look for patterns of behavior and what is happening at those times. For example, the behavior may occur more often in a shower than in a tub bath or when there are two caregivers but not when there is one. You are uncovering clues to factors or triggers that might be affecting the behavior. You may need to make a "best guess" about possible causes of behavior because a clear cause may not emerge. When looking for causes of behaviors it is helpful to think of four general areas that need to be assessed:

- **Personal factors:** those individual physical and emotional factors such as pain, cold, physical illness or limitations, level of dementia, fear, or need for control

Behavior Tracking Log

Name _____   Date _____

1. When	When does it happen? (e.g., when water is turned on)	
2. What	What is the person doing? (e.g., hitting, biting)	
3. Where	Where did the behavior occur? (e.g., in the shower but not in the tub)	
4. Who	Who else was present? What were they doing?	
5. What	What happens before? After?	
6. What	What makes it better? Worse?	

FIGURE 3.1   Behavior tracking log.

- **Relationship factors:** how you relate to the person and his/her unique needs and how the person relates to you
- **Physical environment:** those physical features of the bathing environment such as room temperature and comfort of equipment
- **Organizational environment:** administrative policies and procedures that impact the caregiver's time, approach, flexibility, creativity, and work routines.

Learn the Personal Needs and Capabilities of the Person You Are Bathing

Personal needs can be expressed both verbally and nonverbally. Observation of what is happening when behaviors occur can uncover the triggers of behavioral symptoms. Common concerns expressed by persons being bathed include being in pain, being cold, and feeling a lack of control, anxiety or fear. Table 3.1 illustrates the many ways these concerns may be expressed.

The most common personal causes of distress are related to physical needs, emotional needs or dementia-related problems.

Physical needs include:

- *Pain:* It is important to look for sources of unnecessary or excess disability caused by untreated pain. What physical handicaps does the person have? Is he/she stiff? Does he/she have contractures (limited range of motion)? Other common causes of pain during bathing include: sensitive skin, sensitive feet, stroke-related pain, and arthritis. Refer to chapter 6 for a more detailed discussion of pain.
- *Acute illnesses:* A change in physical health can trigger agitation or aggression. Look for signs of delirium. These include:
  - Difficulty shifting or sustaining attention
  - Stupor or decreased level of consciousness
  - Tactile and/or auditory hallucinations

TABLE 3.1 Ways Common Concerns May Be Expressed During Bathing

	Pain	Feeling Lack of Control	Anxiety/Fear	Cold
Verbal/ Vocal	Says: "That hurts." Asks to "stop" Repeatedly asks for help Complains Moans and groans Screams and yells Mutters in a distressed tone Swears Unusual noise he/she makes intensifies in volume and in pitch Cries	Says: "No!" Threatens, curses, and insults Makes demands Screams and yells Says "Why are you doing this to me?"	Screams and yells Calls for help from others: a spouse, friend, the police, 911 Calls out in pain before being touched Says "You're going to kill me."	Says: "I'm cold!" Says: "I'm hot!" Yells and screams
Nonverbal	Winces Grimaces Flinches Rubs area Guards area Fidgets, repositions self Generalized tension Pulls away or other avoidance behaviors Extreme facial expressions Restlessness Rocks Rigidity Clenches fist Slow movements Noisy breathing Hits Bites	Pulls away, pushes away Hits, bites, and grabs Scowls Spits and scratches Refuses to enter bathroom Points finger at caregiver Attempts to leave	Rigidity Grabs Worried/fearful expression Clenches fist Wrings hands Jittery Shivers Withdraws from caregiver touch	Shivers Tries to cover self Cold hands and feet Trembling lips

19

- Disturbed sleep/wake cycle
- Fluctuations in symptoms.

A sudden change in behavior is often your first clue to physical illness in a person who cannot communicate discomfort verbally. Watch for other signs of acute illness such as lethargy, agitation, increased temperature, or congestion.

- *Cold:* As individuals age, many become sensitive to cold. Once a person is cold, it takes longer to warm up. Clues that a person is cold are: complaints about the temperature of the room or water, shivering, and efforts to cover up.

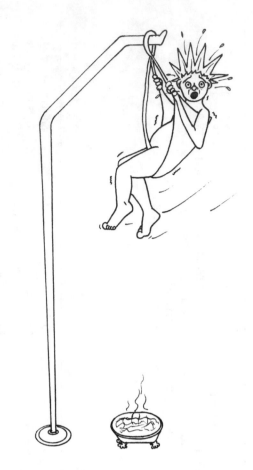

FIGURE 3.2   Fearful experience of the lift.

Look for Signs of Untreated Pain or Illness

Mrs. Gross cries throughout her bath. Efforts to comfort her or change her bathing routine do not help. Staff report that she has recently begun pacing up and down the halls, mumbling continuously in an agitated manner. This mumbling becomes louder and develops into crying anytime someone tries to assist her with dressing or eating.

Discussion: *Mrs. Gross's behavior was triggered by a new, undiagnosed medical problem. Because of her dementia she could not tell anyone that she was in pain. She could only mumble and cry. Since this was not normal behavior for her, a physical exam was performed, and a bowel obstruction discovered. The obstruction caused a great deal of pain and, consequently, her crying. Thus, it was not the bathing technique that was the problem, but an expression of an unmet physical need.*

Emotional needs include:

- *Feeling safe and secure:* There are many factors that can cause the person being bathed to be afraid. Some areas to explore include: fear of falling on transfer, fear of a new caregiver or new bathroom, or unexplained noises in the bathing room. Watch for signals that suggest fear such as a fearful facial expression (wide-open eyes, open or tensed mouth, eyebrows in a straight line), an effort to get away from the caregiver or

bathroom, or a refusal to enter the bathroom or shower area.

- *Freedom from mood or sleep problems:* Depression can be difficult to diagnose in persons with dementia. However, untreated depression can cause emotional pain. Look for the following signs of depression: sleep disturbance, poor appetite, restlessness, irritability, complaints of tiredness, worthlessness or guilt, and lack of interest in other things or people. If the person is depressed, is he/she on an antidepressant and a large enough dose to decrease symptoms?
- *Respect for beliefs about modesty:* Many elderly persons have never been comfortable being naked. Watch for efforts to keep covered or exclamations of concern when private areas are uncovered or touched.
- *Feeling of a sense of control:* All persons need to feel that they have control over what happens

to them. When a person loses even the ability to control when and how they will be touched, undressed, or washed, it is devastating. This is often expressed in demands, threats, or refusal to cooperate.

Dementia-related problems: People with Alzheimer's disease and related problems often develop symptoms to which the caregiver must adjust. Often, as the dementing disease progresses, a person is unable to understand what is happening or communicate needs. Changes in the person's mental and functional abilities may be subtle and occur over time. How this occurs varies from person to person. However, organizing these changes into the three stages of Alzheimer's disease can sometimes be helpful in understanding the disease and are summarized in Table 3.2.

Often different kinds of behavioral symptoms arise at different stages of dementia. For example, a mildly demented person is more likely to verbally refuse a bath by saying: "I've already had a bath." Persons with moderate dementia may say "Stop!" when you approach the bathroom or hold firmly to the doorjamb and refuse to enter the bathroom. Severely demented persons may moan or cry when they enter the bathroom. Examples of dementia-related behaviors as well as possible strategies for addressing them are in Table 3.3.

When assessing a person's strengths and dementia-related problems, get answers to the following questions:

- How does the person communicate? Is he/she able to tell you what is wrong? Can he/she understand simple words or do you need to use gestures and physical guidance to help the person understand?
- What problems does the person have with impulse control, judgment, and understanding events or interactions?
- How is the person's hearing and vision? Is there an impairment that may contribute to a lack of understanding?
- Can the person do routine tasks without assistance? How much help is needed? (See chapter 5 for a detailed discussion of the assessment of the appropriate level of assistance.)

TABLE 3.2 Possible Characteristics of Persons With Mild, Moderate, and Severe Dementia

	Mild	Moderate	Severe
Orientation	Some disorientation to time	Oriented to name only	Disoriented in all spheres
Memory	Fluctuations— Unable to recall some major, old information and learn new information	Can recognize familiar people Largely unaware of recent events Sketchy knowledge of past life Generally unaware of surroundings/seasons	No recognizable memory
ADLs	No assistance needed with toileting and eating, some with choosing proper clothing	Needs some assistance with all ADLs Becomes incontinent	Totally dependent
Behavior/Personality	Some changes: apathetic, some suspiciousness	Repetitive, obsessive behaviors; irritability; fidgety; psychosis; sleep disturbances	Extreme irritability
Problem Solving/ Judgment	Impaired planning and decision making	Severely impaired: unable to understand limitations or consequences of actions	No discernible ability, unable to problem solve
Language	Word finding problems	Language usually becomes "word salad" as disease progresses	All verbal abilities lost
Mobility	Unimpaired	Ambulatory until end of this stage; may be restless	Unable to walk, sit, or (eventually) hold up head
Attention	Slightly reduced	Easily distracted and some trouble starting or stopping task	Severely impaired
Perception	Mild problems in new areas	Unable to recognize common objects and environmental cues	Severely impaired

TABLE 3.3 Dementia-Related Behaviors

Cognitive Skill	Example	Action
Memory	Person tells you she already had a bath	Avoid arguing or reasoning
	Failure to recognize caregiver	Use the same caregiver every day
	Person stops during a bathing step	Gently remind person of next step
Language Communication	Unable to understand what others say	Keep it simple
		Use gestures or modeling
		Keep your body language open and friendly
		Use visual props and cues to augment words
		Match your words and body language
		Make frequent eye contact if culturally appropriate
	Unable to put thoughts into words	Anticipate the person's needs
		Give the person your undivided attention
Perception Problems	Failure to recognize objects such as washcloth or soap	Hand the person the object and use physical guidance to show how to use it
		Explain every step
	Misinterprets environmental cues and has difficulty adjusting to new places	Use frequent reassurance
		Keep environment stable
	Inability to judge depth such as that of the tub, afraid to step over the side	If the person seems to be afraid of falling, give extra support and reassurance
Motor Functioning	Inability to perform spontaneous movements	Explain every step, use physical guidance
	Inability to stop or start a task	Use physical guidance to help the person get started
		Use distraction to stop repetitive actions
Judgment	Accuses caregivers of interfering and refuses to cooperate with requests	Try to anticipate problem areas
		Avoid confrontation
		Stop at the first sign of negative emotion and try to figure out what is going on
	Responds to requests with fear and anxiety	Explain what you are doing at all times and avoid surprises
		Limit choices
Attention	Short attention span and easily distracted	Repeat verbal prompts
		Use touch to get the person's attention
		Give simple one-step instructions
		Never leave the person unattended in the bath or shower
		Make eye contact
		Eliminate distractions
Body Orientation	Unable to identify body parts	Use gestures (pointing and motioning)
		Use physical guidance when gesturing
		Give simple verbal prompts
	Unable to understand the difference between right and left	Avoid instructions such as "raise your right arm"
		Use verbal prompts along with touch

Additional content contributed by C. G. Rapp, V. Shue, and C. Beck.

Adapting to Personal Factors

When Mrs. Peters was invited to bathe by Paula, her caregiver, she would shake her fist and threaten Paula. She would shout that she had already had her bath and that she wanted to be left alone. Mrs. Peters was in the early stages of dementia. Her language skills were good, and she could bathe herself, but her memory and judgment were poor. Her bath time was usually around 10 a.m. after she had already dressed for the day and had her breakfast. She did not remember that she had not had a bath and did not realize that she was dirty. Trying to convince her only made matters worse and she would become more insistent that she had already taken a bath.

Discussion: Several personal factors are triggering Mrs. Peters' aggressive response. These include both dementia-related factors and needing to feel a sense of control. To adapt to both, Paula avoided arguing with her. She approached Mrs. Peters before she had dressed and chatted with her about her farm duties, using information she knew about her personal history. Once she had established rapport with Mrs. Peters, Paula asked her if she would like to get ready for her day. Mrs. Peters responded yes, went willingly to the shower room, and washed herself. A battle was avoided as Paula found a way to give Mrs. Peters a sense of control and use her remaining skills. She never mentioned the word bath but used Mrs. Peters' language of "getting ready for the day." Mrs. Peters viewed Paula's invitation to the bath as questioning her judgment. Mrs. Peters was offended by the suggestion that she was dirty and hadn't cleaned herself, so she felt she had to defend herself. Paula also took the time to create a friendly, validating relationship by talking with Mrs. Peters about the things she used to do on her farm.

Consider Relationship/Interpersonal Factors

Your behavior can often unknowingly trigger distress. When you become aware of the effect of your behaviors and change your approach, behavioral symptoms often decrease. Pay particular attention to your own nonverbal messages. They are conveyed through tone of voice, facial expressions, and gestures, which often communicate more than words. Be sure your nonverbal messages match your words and convey caring. Answer the following questions to determine what interpersonal factors might be contributing to the person's distress.

- Do you repeatedly respond to complaints of pain or cold, apologize and take some action? (Persons with dementia may not process or remember your responses and need frequent repetitions.)
- Are there too many people in the bathroom? Could this be overwhelming?
- Are you talking with someone else in the room or focused on the person being bathed? Are you using a friendly, calm approach with good eye contact, if culturally appropriate?
- Do you explain each step in simple language and match your communication to the person's abilities?
- Do you smile often?
- Are you moving too fast for this person?
- Are you trying to do too much at one time?
- Do you acknowledge and respect the person's need for privacy?
- Do you consider gender preferences?

Focusing on the Relationship

Mrs. Johns resisted bathing. Her caregiver, Rose, learned from Mrs. Johns' family that she had loved to shop. Rose brought in a catalogue for Mrs. Johns to look at while she was being washed with a no-rinse soap and water. She would ask Mrs. Johns what she liked best on each page and created a fun experience for both of them. Whenever Mrs. Johns complained, Rose would apologize and take action to correct the complaint.

Discussion: Rose has a positive, interpersonal approach. She is very good at focusing on the person she is bathing and works to make the bath a pleasurable experience. She makes an effort to get to know the person. She uses personal information about Mrs. Johns to find a way to help distract her from an unpleasant task. Rather than focusing on the washing task, Rose pays close attention to Mrs. Johns's needs. She is quick to apologize and change her approach, if possible. Rose's residents feel connected to her and well cared for.

Caregiver Wisdom

One gentleman was verbally gruff with me the first few times I bathed him. But I developed a comfortable, consistent routine for him; he saw that I cared about how he felt. Also, I always explained to him what we were doing. He became very cooperative and pleasant. After the fourth bath, he told his wife I was so good that I needed a raise in pay! That made me feel good. That is a success story.

Debbie Medina, CNA, Hood River
Care Center, Hood River, OR

Assess for Stressful Factors in the Physical Environment

Areas to explore in the physical environment include:

- **Lighting:** Is there enough lighting for an older person's eyes? Is it nonglare? Does the person squint when entering the bathroom?
- **Temperature:** Is the room warm enough? Is the person shivering or trying to stay covered? Are there complaints of cold? Is there a heat lamp in the bathing room?
- **Seating and mobility devices:** Is the equipment comfortable and fitted to the person? Does the person cry out or wince when placed on the shower chair? Does the person squirm in the shower chair, lean to the side or make attempts to get up? Does the person's bottom sink into the hole in the shower chair? Are the person's legs supported? Is the person frightened when placed on a lift?
- **Space:** Is the area cluttered with extra equipment, making it frightening or difficult to maneuver?

- **Noise level:** Can you hear unpleasant or unusual noises when you're in the bathroom? Is the person disturbed by these noises? Does the running water make conversation difficult? Is the person having difficulty hearing you? Do you have pleasant, person-specific music playing, if soothing?
- **Homelike atmosphere:** Is the bathroom institutional looking? Does the person fail to recognize that it is a bathroom? Is there adequate privacy?
- **Odors:** Are there unpleasant odors in the room? Are the room sprays being used pleasant or unpleasant? Does the person seem to be reacting to them?

Assessing Physical Factors

Mrs. Smith is a thin, frail 93-year-old with a history of hip fracture, arthritis, and peripheral neuropathy. When the typical plastic shower chair with the large hole and no foot support is used, her bottom sinks in the chair, causing pressure on her fractured hip and arthritic joints. Her legs hang as deadweight, and her feet turn blue as she complains bitterly of pain in her bottom, hip, and legs.

<u>Discussion:</u> Mrs. Smith is a good example of factors in the physical environment being the cause of her discomfort. The room is cold and the equipment does not fit her body, which triggers her complaints. She needs a more comfortable seating device, a footstool, and extra covering to keep her warm. When a child's padded potty-seat insert is placed in the shower chair, her feet are supported on a small stool, and she is well covered, her complaints decrease dramatically.

Assess the Organizational Environment

Rigid administrative policies and practices can hamper your ability to provide individualized care. Assess the following areas for possible triggers of discomfort:

- **Philosophy:** Does the philosophy of care allow for flexibility in determining when, how, and who

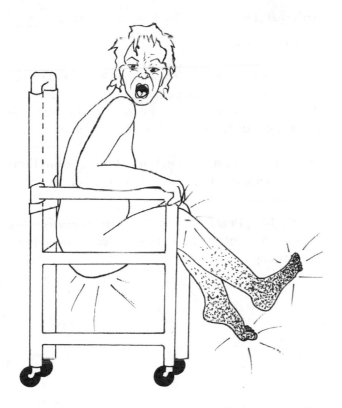

FIGURE 3.3 Mrs. Smith in poorly fitting, uncomfortable shower chair.

will be bathed? When persons are distressed, are you criticized if you postpone some tasks and clean only the essential areas?

- **Policies and procedures:** Is there a policy that dictates the frequency and types of baths? Can you substitute a bed bath for a shower?
- **Supervision and staffing patterns:** How many different caregivers might bathe a person each month? Do staffing patterns support individualized care? Are caregivers rotated among groups so that they do not care for the same person every day? Are there consistent assignments so direct caregivers get to know the people they care for?
- **Structure of the day:** Are all baths expected to be done in the morning? Are staff on all shifts encouraged to adjust when baths are given to meet the habits and preferences of individuals?
- **Staff support and education:** Does the training and supervision of nursing assistants teach a rigid procedure for showering or reinforce the use of flexibility and individualization? What strategies for coping with agitation and aggression are

taught? Is distress during bathing considered normal for persons with dementia or seen as a need for further assessment and intervention?

- **Equipment and supplies:** Is there a wide variety of bathing supplies available to meet individual needs? Is there a limit to the supplies that can be used for one bath?

Rigid Rules

Mrs. Jones is a 60-year-old woman with mild dementia. She refuses to shower and is able to state that she "doesn't like a shower." She cannot elaborate on her reasons but she is adamant in her refusal. The nursing home where she resides requires two showers a week. She must be forced to shower, resulting in self-protective behaviors such as hitting and kicking. Sometimes it takes four staff members to shower her. This is very upsetting to all involved.

Discussion: Mrs. Jones illustrates the problems caused by rigid policies. When the two showers a week rule is discontinued, alternative methods of bathing can be tried. An in-bed towel bath was tried and Mrs. Jones responded very favorably to this change. She called it her "steam bath," and she smiled and was very cooperative. She was clean and happy. Finding ways to meet the individual needs of persons with dementia requires flexibility.

SUMMARY

A behavior such as yelling can have many causes and will respond to different solutions depending upon whether the cause is personal, interpersonal, environmental, or a combination of factors. If you think the person's distress is caused by cold, you can begin by assessing for personal factors such as decreased body fat, a history of sensitivity to cold, or circulatory problems. Next, assess the environment. Check the temperature in the room. Also, look at how you respond to the person's behavior. Do you try to keep him/her covered? Do you acknowledge complaints of cold?

Understanding the causes or triggers for behavioral symptoms that occur during bathing is the first step in stopping the bathing battle. This helps you to tailor your approach to the individual needs of the person you are bathing. Gather as much information as you can about the person. Then select one behavior that suggests that the person is uncomfortable. Look for the trigger(s) for this behavior by assessing the physical, emotional, and dementia-related needs of the person, the quality of the interaction during the bath, and the characteristics of the physical and organizational environments. The information gathered will guide you in selecting the solutions to improve the bathing experience.

APPENDIX
PERSONAL HISTORY

The forms on the following pages can be used to gather information to help you understand behavior and develop bathing routines that are tailored to meet the unique needs of each individual. They include:

- **Personal Information Data Sheet:** Use this form for helpful information about the person's past and current life.

- **Bathing Preferences and Practices Form:** This can be sent to the family to learn about prior bathing habits.

Personal Information Data Sheet

Name _____

Nickname _____

Occupation _____

Past Accomplishments _____

Education _____

Current Interests/Activities _____

Hobbies, topics of interest _____

Family: Spouse   Yes ☐ No ☐   Name _____

        Children   Yes ☐ No ☐   Names _____

Other regular visitors _____

Favorite Foods _____

Favorite Music _____

Level of Dementia

    Able to understand words?   Yes ☐   No ☐

    Able to remember _____ Family _____ Caregiver _____ Events

    Difficulty with judgment   Yes ☐   No ☐

    Able to help with bath   Yes ☐   No ☐

    Able to signal toileting needs   Yes ☐   No ☐   If no, how do you know his/her toileting needs?

_____

Personality _____

Current medical problems _____

Pain site, if any

_____ back _____ hips _____ feet _____ head

Other (where?) _____

Spiritual beliefs/religion _____

Cultural beliefs/prejudices _____

Language _____

Summary from Bathing Preferences Form _____

_____

_____

FIGURE 3.4   Personal information data sheet.

Bathing Preferences and Practices Form

In order to better care for _____,
we would like to learn about his/her bathing history and preferences. We would appreciate you providing as much information as possible.

Your name: _____

Relationship to resident: _____'s

The following questions are about _____ bathing habits. Please describe his/her habits both before the disease and after by checking one box in the "before illness" column and one in the "after illness" column.

1. How many times each week did he/she bathe?

Before	Illness		After	Illness
☐	☐	less than once/week		
☐	☐	1-2 times/wk		
☐	☐	3-4 times/wk		
☐	☐	more than 4 times/wk		

2. What time of day did he/she bathe? (Check all that apply)

Before	Illness		After	Illness
☐	☐	before 7 a.m.		
☐	☐	morning		
☐	☐	afternoon		
☐	☐	evening		
☐	☐	just before bed		

3. How long was his/her bath?

Before	Illness		After	Illness
☐	☐	less than 10 minutes		
☐	☐	15-30 minutes		
☐	☐	30-60 minutes		
☐	☐	more than 1 hour		

4. Where did he/she bathe?

Before	Illness		After	Illness
☐	☐	bathtub		
☐	☐	shower		
☐	☐	sponge bath		

5. Which bathing items were used? (check all that apply)

☐ wash cloth
☐ sponge
☐ brush
☐ special soap (what kind?): _____
☐ other (describe): _____

6. Describe the way he/she rinsed the soap:

☐ with water from the shower nozzle
☐ with remaining bath water in tub
☐ using a bathside commode/basin
☐ other (describe): _____

7. Did he/she use talcum powder after bathing?

____ No   ____ Yes (what kind): _____

8. Did he/she use moisturizing lotion?

____ No   ____ Yes (what kind): _____

9. Describe his/her feeling about bathing in general?

Before	Illness		After	Illness
☐	☐	strongly dislikes		
☐	☐	mildly dislikes		
☐	☐	neutral		
☐	☐	likes		
☐	☐	strongly likes		

10. How was bathing started (after illness began)?

☐ he/she started it by himself/herself
☐ you suggested it once
☐ you suggested it several times
☐ only by physically bringing him/her to the bathing area

FIGURE 3.5   Bathing preferences and practices form.

The following questions are about _____'s ability to bathe himself/herself immediately before admission. Please describe the help you or another caregiver provided, if any.

1. Describe his/her ability to get undressed for the bath:

   ☐ He/she needs no help
   ☐ Undressed self with encouragement
   ☐ You helped with less than half of the undressing
   ☐ You did it all

2. Did you prepare the bath for him/her (turn on water to fill a basin)?

   _____ No   _____ Yes

3. Describe his/her ability to get in the bath or shower:

   ☐ He/she needs no help
   ☐ He/she got in with encouragement
   ☐ You helped with less than half
   ☐ You helped with more than half
   ☐ You put him/her in

4. Describe his/her ability to wash herself:

   ☐ He/she needs no help
   ☐ Undressed self with encouragement
   ☐ You helped with less than half the washing
   ☐ You helped with more than half the washing
   ☐ You did it all

5. Describe how he/she dried herself:

   ☐ He/she needs no help
   ☐ He/she dried self with encouragement
   ☐ You helped with less than half the drying
   ☐ You helped with more than half the drying
   ☐ You did it all

6. Describe his/her ability to get dressed after the bath:

   ☐ He/she needs no help
   ☐ He/she dressed self with encouragement
   ☐ You helped with less than half the dressing
   ☐ You helped with more than half the dressing
   ☐ You did it all

Your answers to the following will help us find ways to make bathing a safer, easier, and more enjoyable activity for all residents and staff. Please give as much information as you can.

1. Please tell us about any problems you faced while bathing (undressing, getting in and out of the tub, washing, drying, or dressing).

2. Can you give us any "special tips" which you found helpful in bathing? Please describe all the things you did or said that helped make the bathing process easier and more pleasurable either for you or him/her.

Thank you very much for taking time to answer these questions

Developed by S. Dwyer, A. L. Barrick, and P. D. Sloane (University of North Carolina at Chapel Hill) as part of the research grant, Reducing Disruptive Behaviors in Dementia During Bathing (R01 AG1150E), funded by the National Institute on Aging. This form may be reproduced for clinical, research, or teaching purposes.

FIGURE 3.5 Bathing preferences and practices form. (*continued*)

CHAPTER 4

Selecting Individualized Solutions That Work

Ann Louise Barrick, Joanne Rader,
and Madeline Mitchell

To increase comfort during the bath, you need to develop a realistic, individualized care plan that addresses the personal needs, preferences and abilities identified in your assessment. In addition, you may need to modify the environment. All this requires thought and planning. Following the assessment, there are two steps to this thoughtful process: selecting and then testing solutions. You can use the Intervention Planning Table (see chapter appendix) as a tool to help you develop and try out your plan. Photocopy and place it in the person's flowchart. It will help you and other caregivers know what new solutions have been tried, how they have worked, and new ideas to try.

Set Realistic Expectations

For most people with dementia, the goal of making bathing pleasurable or at least tolerable is realistic. For others, bathing is extremely upsetting and only small improvements in comfort are possible. For these individuals the best you can do is provide some distraction and a slight decrease in discomfort. For example, we worked with one woman who yelled and tried to hit the caregiver every time she was touched. We tried different kinds of baths and interventions. We found that only distraction and a very gentle, slow, supportive approach, stopping every time she started to yell or strike at us seemed to help. We could distract her by having her hold and comfort a doll and using a second caregiver to talk with her. With these efforts we were able to clean her and slightly decrease the discomfort expressed by yelling and hitting.

Establish the Goals for the Bath

In addition to the general goal that you want the bath to be more pleasurable, you need to identify and select one specific behavior to address. Does the person yell? Hit? Try to bite? How often does this happen? Identify changes in behavior that will let you know that the person is less distressed. You can define your goal in terms of a reduction in behavioral symptoms and/or an increase in signs of pleasure. Will it be a decrease in complaints of being cold from 7–10 per bath to less than 3 per bath? Will it be a decrease in the percentage of time the person makes a wailing noise during bathing? Will the best measure be an increase in the number of times the person smiles during the shower or the fact that he smiles at all? Table 4.1 gives some examples of various goals and how to measure them.

For example, we worked with a gentleman who always cried out whenever we tried to wash him. He had been a minister and liked to sing. Anytime he began to yell, his caregiver stopped what she was doing, quieted her tone, used gentle touch, and asked him if he would sing a hymn for her. The singing calmed his anxieties, distracted him, and created a way for him to be of service to others. The more he sang the less he yelled! This was a good measure of success.

If a person becomes distressed when being bathed you have to ask yourself what really needs to be cleaned now. What areas are dirty? What tasks can be done at another time? For example, hair washing can be very distressing. If the person's hair does not look greasy, it is best to postpone that task until another day. In another example, Mrs. Brown was upset just at the mention of the word "bath." The usual routine was to shower, wash her hair, cut her toenails and fingernails, and brush her teeth all as part of the same bathing experience. She became increasingly upset during the course of this "bath." She began by saying no, then started to cry, and then escalated to trying to hit her caregiver. When her hair, nails, and teeth were done at a different time, there was a noticeable improvement in her comfort level as shown by a reduction in complaints and elimination of the hitting behavior. The routine of getting it all done at once was altered to avoid the battle.

Determine the Level of Independence

Can this person do any part of the bath himself? What level of assistance is needed to maximize independence and minimize unnecessary disability? Involving the person in the bath and having him/her wash those parts he/she can, may help to make the bath more pleasurable. However, encouraging independence in someone unable to perform a task may increase agitation. Understanding the level of dementia and specific deficits will help you select strategies that fit the person's abilities. During the course of our study, as the nursing assistant developed a relationship with the person, we were often surprised by the emergence of previously hidden abilities to do self-care such as washing one's own face, chest, and "private parts," even in persons who were severely impaired. Different techniques seem to work better depending on the person's level of dementia. For example, the milder the dementia, the more useful are the techniques of talking with the person, asking him/her to help, or giving choices. See chapter 5 for a detailed discussion of methods for choosing the best level of assistance.

Persons in the later stages of dementia tend to respond well to physical guidance and distractions such as something to hold, look at, or eat or drink. Of course, it is essential when working with persons with dementia to assess if they are likely to try to place objects in their mouths that could cause choking. When you are providing food or drink, be aware of swallowing and dietary precautions, and make choices that are pleasing to the individual, but also safe.

Determine the Level of Communication to Use

What can the person understand? It is important to use the person's vocabulary. If the person uses the word "poop" to describe having a bowel movement, that is the word you should use when talking to him/her. Adapt your communication style to the person's level of understanding. For example, use verbal interventions with a person who can understand simple language. Nonverbal interventions such as food or other distracting objects are helpful with a person with more advanced dementia. Examples of distracters are in Table 4.2.

Select Solutions That Meet Specific Needs

Your job is to fit the solution to the person. Choose strategies that address the possible causes of the behav-

TABLE 4.1   Setting Measurable Goals

Behaviors	Goal	How Measured
Distressed Behaviors		
Pinching	Reduce by 50%	Decrease pinching from 6 times per bath to 3 by (date)
Crying out	Reduce by 75%	Decrease episodes from 20 to 5 per bath
Screams when bottom washed	No screaming	Record if screaming did or did not occur during task
Positive Behaviors		
Engaging in conversation	Respond to questions	Will respond to at least 2 questions per bath
Sings with caregiver	Person will sing when caregiver initiates, showing an increase in comfort	Person will sing once per bath from current once per 4 baths
Thanks caregiver	Person will be comfortable during bathing	He/she expresses appreciation for help. Smiles, laughs, or hugs caregiver during 3 consecutive baths.

ioral symptoms. Because behaviors are so complicated and can have different triggers, you often have to try many different things to discover what makes the person the most comfortable. For example, if the person appears to be cold (yells, grabs clothing as you try to remove it) you can use both environmental and interpersonal solutions. Try warming the room before bringing the person to the bathing room. When the person complains of being cold, cover him/her, apologize, and reassure him/her that you will make every effort to keep him/her warm. At other times you may want to try one solution at a time. For example, if the person appears to be afraid of falling you may begin by reassuring him/her often in a calm, soothing voice. Next you can try using a different type of transfer (see chapter 8). If this does not decrease his/her distress, you may want to try a bed bath instead of a shower to eliminate the trigger for his/her fear.

Caregiver Wisdom

Finding a reason can really make a difference. You can't force anyone! One person who hates a shower will take a bath if I catch her in a good mood and then talk about her husband. I say: "He likes it when you smell so good!" Then when we're in the shower I make her feel special because she likes to be waited on.

Angell Neal, CNA, Brian Center of Clayton, Clayton, NC

You may think that pain is the cause of a person's yelling. You know his/her feet are very sensitive and he/she seems to yell most when you are washing them.

You may want to wash his/her feet last so as not to upset him/her. Or you can try soaking his/her feet first to loosen dirt and gently use the edge of a baby washcloth to wash between the toes. Apologize at any sign of pain.

Success usually requires great creativity and persistence. It may take 3–4 weeks before finding the right combination of solutions. There is no "cookbook" for bathing. Each solution must be carefully selected. Music can provide distraction and relaxation. But you have to know and use very specific types of music with each person—country western for some, classical for others. Similarly, food and objects you choose for the person to hold or look at need to be selected based on your knowledge of the person, and trial and error. The following case study illustrates this process.

Case Study

Mrs. Swanson did not enjoy her routine showers. She often said she did not want to go, and almost constantly cried and complained of pain and being cold. She asked staff to hurry up. Sometimes she mixed words up, saying, for example, that the water was too hot when she really meant too cold.

Before helping her, we (Rader and the nursing assistant) reviewed what we knew or could locate in the chart about her. She was 93-years-old and very proud of having been a preacher's wife. She also made women's hats and liked fashion. She had been very active in the church, and her beliefs remained a source of support for her. She had done a lot of handwork, such as embroidery, and enjoyed cooking and baking. She had entered the nursing home 2 years before after fracturing her hip. Her diagnoses included Alzheimer's dis-

TABLE 4.2   Sample Distracters

Food	Conversation	Objects to Hold	Others
Cookies	About family	A towel	Music
Gum	About food	A washcloth	A balloon to observe
Crackers	About pets	A stuffed animal	A plant to observe
Lollipop	About the farm	Your hand	A mobile
Bananas	About past work	A small figurine	
Peppermints	How attractive they are	A sponge	
Chocolate	Ask questions	A ball	
Coffee	Ask opinions	A mirror	
Tea	Give praise	A doll	
Cake			

ease, arthritis, peripheral neuropathy (from diabetes), and limited vision and hearing. She was incontinent of both urine and stool.

Her history included many possible sources of pain—arthritis, previous hip fracture, peripheral neuropathy, and some, as yet undiagnosed, illness. We noted that Mrs. Swanson had an order for acetaminophen four times a day as necessary for pain, but that she rarely received it.

As we began to work with her, we tried to view the bath from her perspective. We noticed that she was transferred using a two-person underarm assist, and that during this process her face was anxious, and she complained of pain. In the bathroom, we noticed that the bathing chair was a standard one, made of plastic pipe with a hard seat, and that the room temperature was cool. After this initial assessment, we felt her major sources of distress came from her needs for comfort, warmth, and security.

Based on this assessment, we focused on trying to reduce pain and increase warmth. We asked that the acetaminophen be given routinely and made sure that she got a dose early in the morning, so that it would be working by the time we assisted her in the shower. We cushioned the shower chair with a padded seat and warmed the shower room by turning on the heat lamp before bringing her in. We kept her covered with towels while showering, lifting the towels to wash small areas, and rinsed her body with a handheld nozzle. In addition, we played church music in an effort to distract and relax her, though it was difficult to know how much she understood because of her hearing loss and the fact that the music echoed in the bathroom.

Her complaints decreased, but the shower was not yet a pleasant experience for her. So we renewed our efforts and tried some other things. We asked that she be given additional pain medication (a narcotic) prior to the shower. But her pain complaints, mostly related to being moved, did not change; and the medication only made her drowsy. Looking again at the physical environment, we decided to no longer use the handheld shower to rinse her, since the water spray seemed to trigger and increase her discomfort and her leg pain. So we started washing her with baby washcloths, using a no-rinse soap solution in a basin, and kept her covered and warm the entire time, lifting the towels to wash.

At the same time, the nursing assistant experimented with techniques of distraction when Mrs. Swanson appeared anxious. They sang hymns together, "The Old Rugged Cross" being a favorite. She gave Mrs. Swanson small plastic figurines to hold and comment on, or talked about her son or her work in the church. This worked well when used just before a difficult procedure such as washing her buttocks and underside. Before the nursing assistant touched an area that might be painful, she also told Mrs. Swanson she was going to touch her and that she would be careful. If Mrs. Swanson complained of pain or being cold, the nursing assistant would apologize and take some action to address her need, such as covering an area or readjusting her in the shower chair. We also soaked her feet in a basin of water while we washed her in the shower, and she found this soothing.

To help make transfers less painful, we consulted with a physical therapist who suggested trying a sliding board transfer, going slow, and explaining the moves step-by-step. This decreased Mrs. Swanson's complaints slightly. Our "best guess" was that fear and anxiety were also playing a role, so we added new solutions. We asked her to count with us before we started the transfer; this yielded fewer complaints of pain and fear.

A surprisingly effective intervention during the shower was to give her a mirror to hold. The nursing assistant thought of this, remembering that Mrs. Swanson always looked in the hall mirror when she was wheeled down the hall. As Mrs. Swanson held the mirror, the nursing assistant would comment about how nice she was going to look after the bath.

Because Mrs. Swanson disliked having her hair washed, we did this last, taking care to keep her warm and well covered. We wet her head with washcloths, using minimal shampoo. We carefully poured from a small graduated pitcher, avoiding her face and ears. This, along with talking with her pleasantly about topics of interest, made the hair washing more pleasant for her. At the same time, we shared simple jokes with her, and sometimes we could get her to laugh.

This was a trial and error process. The result was an individualized bathing care plan that worked for Mrs. Swanson (Table 4.3). Measurable improvements included the following behaviors:

- She agreed to the shower.
- She no longer cried in the shower.
- Her complaints of pain decreased from 10 per bath to under 5.
- Her complaints of being cold decreased from 15 per bath to under 3.

TABLE 4.3 Individualized Shower Care Plan for Mrs. Swanson

Needs Identified:

For comfort—has pain particularly in her legs and feet
To be warm
To feel safe

Behavioral Symptoms:

Crying, complaints of being cold, in pain
Refusing shower

Goals:

Increase comfort related to transfers and foot and leg pain
Decrease fear and anxiety and increase pleasure
Keep her warm

Suggested Approaches:

To increase comfort and warmth:
- Give routine Tylenol 1 hour before shower
- Shower before breakfast
- Assess her level of discomfort before you begin
- Turn on heat lamp in shower room to warm it
- Pad shower chair with child potty-seat insert
- Move her carefully and slowly
- Tell her before you touch her, especially her feet; touch legs gently and move legs up and down gently before beginning transfer
- Use sliding board transfer
- Go slowly and ask her to count with you before transfer
- Use touch and soothing voice to reassure her you care and understand that she hurts
- Position carefully in shower chair
- Keep her well covered throughout shower, lifting towel to wash areas; use basin with washcloths and no-rinse soap solution instead of water spray
- Sincerely apologize if she complains of pain, being cold
- Try singing hymns with her
- Distract her with objects such as a hand mirror, cute figurines

To decrease fear and anxiety:

- Distract her with conversation on favorite topics—her son, her, the church
- Speak clearly and distinctly, making eye contact as much as possible so she can read lips
- Explain any misunderstanding she has related to being hard of hearing (e.g., She hears "watch" instead of "wash")
- Respond quickly to her complaints of being cold by adding blankets, etc.
- Wash hair last—be sure she is warm and well covered with bath blanket before beginning; wet head with washcloths; use a small amount of baby shampoo; rinse using small amount of water from small pitcher, deflecting water from face and ears.

- She showed interest in objects she was holding.
- She would thank the nursing assistant for her help.

Reaching these goals took getting to know Mrs. Swanson, viewing the shower through her eyes, modifying the environment, and meeting her needs for comfort and security. This required ongoing thinking and planning, but the final result took no additional time for the nursing assistant and was much more pleasant for Mrs. Swanson.

Try a Bedbath

It has only been in the last 60–80 years that indoor plumbing, bathtubs, and showers have been commonplace, yet people have been getting clean for centuries. History illustrates that there are many ways to get clean. In-bed bathing is one. The bed bath is often a good choice for persons who are frail, nonambulatory, experience pain with transfers, or are fearful of lifts. In addition, persons who are considerably overweight often enjoy having the option of a bed bath to avoid the use of lifts and possible embarrassment in the shower. For these individuals it is also sometimes easier to wash skin folds when the person is lying flat in bed.

The bed bath is usually done with a basin of water, soap and washcloths, and rinsing off the soap. A variation on this method is the towel bath, first described as the Totman Towel Bath Technique. Here the person is covered with a large, warm, moist towel containing a no-rinse soap solution and is washed and massaged through the towel. Dirt and oil are absorbed and removed by the towel and the person is cleaned without rinsing. The person is warm and covered throughout the bath. It is easily adapted to meet individual preferences. Instructions for the towel bath are in Table 4.4. Suggestions for individualizing the towel bath are in Table 4.5.

It is possible to wash people adequately in bed and it is often much less stressful. However, there is a belief about the need to douse or dunk people to get them clean. In some cases the person's skin actually improves (less dry and flaking) when the no-rinse soap method is used in place of a shower. If you have concerns about using a no-rinse method, look for evidence of problems before assuming that a water rinse is necessary. See chapter 7 for a discussion of skin care.

When You Think You've Tried Everything

Sometimes traditional bathing methods, including the towel bath, just don't work. This presents you with a challenge and an opportunity to use your ingenuity and special caregiving skills. Here are some examples of some creative and unique bathing solutions that caregivers have shared:

The recliner bath: Several home health aides have reported giving successful baths when the person is resting in the recliner chair in the living room. They used a basin of water (preferably with a no-rinse soap) and padded each body part being washed with a towel and incontinence pad if available. This worked particularly well for persons fatigued by chronic or terminal illnesses. The goal of a bath or shower is to get the person clean and help him/her feel refreshed. This can be done in many ways. (Note: If the visits are being covered under Medicare, it is important for the aide to "count" this as a bath for reimbursement purposes.)

The commode bath: This method was useful for an easily agitated nursing home resident. Mrs. Harrington disliked being moved or touched and fought through our attempts to carefully shower her or bathe her in bed. She was often incontinent of stool during her morning shower or bath. So the caregiver, Marie, placed her on the toilet in her bathroom, allowed her private time to have a bowel movement, then washed and dressed her upper torso while she sat on the toilet. Next Marie washed her legs and had her stand so she could wash her perineal area and bottom. Her thin hair was washed at the bathroom sink using washcloths to wet and rinse her hair. Marie then transferred her to her wheelchair and she was ready for the day. Some might label it undignified to bathe

TABLE 4.4   The Towel Bath: A Gentle Bed-Bath Method

Equipment:

- 2 or more bath blankets
- 1 large plastic bag containing:
  - 1 large (5'6" x 3') lightweight towel (fanfolded)
  - 1 standard bath towel
  - 2 or more washcloths
- 2–3 quart plastic pitcher filled with water (approximately 105–110° Fahrenheit), to which you have added:
- 1–1 1/2 ounces of no-rinse soap (such as Septa-Soft, manufactured by Calgon-Vestal) (use manufacturer's instructions for dilution)

Preparing the Person:

Explain the bath. Make the room quiet or play soft music. Dim the lights if this calms the person. Assure privacy. Wash hands. If necessary, work one bath blanket under the resident, to protect the linen and provide warmth. Undress the resident, keeping him/her covered with bed linen or the second bath blanket. You may also protect the covering linen by folding it at the end of the bed.

Preparing the Bath:

Pour the soapy water into the plastic bag, and work the solution into the towels and washcloths until they are uniformly damp but not soggy. If necessary, wring out excess solution through the open end of the bag into the sink. Twist the top of the bag closed to retain heat. Take the plastic bag containing the warm towels and washcloths to the bedside.

Bathing the Resident:

Expose the person's feet and lower legs and immediately cover the area with the warm, moist large towel. Then gently and gradually uncover the resident while simultaneously unfolding the wet towel to recover the resident. Place the covers at the end of the bed. Start washing at whatever part of the body is least distressing to the resident. For example, start at the feet and cleanse the body in an upward direction by massaging gently through the towel. You may wish to place a bath blanket over the towel to hold in the warmth. Wash the backs of the legs by bending the person's knee and going underneath. Bathe the face, neck, and ears with one of the washcloths. You may also hand a washcloth to the resident and encourage him to wash his own face. Turn the resident to one side and place the smaller warm towel from the plastic bag on the back, washing in a similar manner, while warming the resident's front with the bath blanket or warm moist towel. No rinsing or drying is required. Use a washcloth from the plastic bag to wash the genital and rectal areas. Gloves should be worn when washing these areas.

After the Bath:

If desired, have the person remain unclothed and covered with the bath blanket and bed linen, dressing at a later time. A dry cotton bath blanket (warmed if possible) placed next to the skin and tucked close provides comfort and warmth. Place used linen back into the plastic bag; tie the bag and place in a hamper.

Adapted with permission from: "Towel Bath—Totman Technique," St. Louis: Calgon-Vestal Laboratories, 1975.

TABLE 4.5   Individualizing the Towel Bath

Change	Explanation
Cover the moist towel with one or two dry bath blankets.	This helps to keep the wet towel warm. For persons who are particularly sensitive to cold, two dry bath blankets increase comfort.
Remove the towel before turning the person over to do his or her back	Some people are more sensitive to cold than others. The wet towel feels cold to them after about 5 minutes.
Do not use a moist towel. Cover the person with a large dry towel and wash under the towel with the washcloths wet with the no-rinse soap mixture.	Some people do not like the wet towel. It feels heavy or "too wet" to them.
Stand to wash back, genital/rectal area, and rectum.	Some persons feel pain when they are being rolled over. Having the person stand saves a painful extra movement. The person will be getting up to get dressed. The key here is to keep the person covered. This can be done with a dry bath blanket or towel.
Double bag the towels with the no-rinse soap mixture.	If the plastic is thin, use two bags; this will help hold in the heat.
Moisten disposable wipes with warm water to wash rectum if it is very soiled.	Wipes tend to be softer and easier to use than a washcloth. The key is to have them warm.
Adjust the light to fit the person's preference (e.g., dim or bright)	Some persons are more relaxed if the lights are low because there are less stimuli. Also, soft lighting and a quiet tone of voice can have a calming effect on the person.

a person while sitting on the toilet, but for Mrs. Harrington, it was the best way to honor her preferences, needs, and abilities.

The singing bath: For another complex person, we tried the singing, sitting, in-room bath. Miss Florence was infamous for refusing her shower and for fighting when she was forced to shower. Estelle, the nursing assistant who worked with her discovered that she liked to sing. Her favorite tunes were "Jesus Loves Me" and "Happy Birthday." If Estelle waited until she felt Miss Florence was in a good mood, sang with her, did part of bath while she was lying in bed and part as she began to get up out of bed (following Miss Florence's lead) she was able to wash her entire body. Her hair was done using an in-bed basin on another day. Interestingly, the family reported that Miss Florence had been refusing to get in the shower or tub for 10 years prior to coming into the care facility.

The waltzing bath: Nina loved shopping and dancing, but hated her shower. Any time staff tried to get her into the shower room, she became resistive and then combative if they persisted. Her nursing assistants came up with an excellent and creative alternative. They placed numerous washcloths in a plastic bag with a warm solution of no-rinse soap. They removed Nina's clothes and covered her with an available poncho-type garment (a bath blanket pinned around the shoulders could also work). One assistant stood in front and began waltzing with Nina and talking about shopping while the other was behind reaching under the cover and washing with the warm, wet, no-rinse washcloths. It was quick and joyful for all.

The seven-day bath: A family reported good luck in keeping their father, Mr. Simmons, clean by dividing the body into seven parts and washing one each day. He disliked bathing or washing but could tolerate short episodes better than longer, more overwhelming ones.

The under-the-clothes bath: Grace disliked the shower and tub, but did well when encouraged to wash herself in her room. However, one day her caregiver, Margaret, arrived to find that Grace had been up all night, which was unusual because she preferred to stay in bed most mornings. She was dressed and sitting in her wheelchair. She had body odor associated with perspiration and urination. A urinary tract infection was suspected and later confirmed and treated. Grace wasn't able to wash herself so Margaret thought she would try to freshen her up and help her feel better. As she talked to Grace about her favorite subjects, she reached under her dress to wash her underarms, breast areas, and genitals. She had her stand briefly so she could wash her rectum. Anytime Grace started to become angry or upset, she stopped to give her time to calm down. It wasn't a complete bath, but the priority areas were cleaned and Margaret avoided a big battle. Sometimes if a person is refusing to remove clothing or holding onto it, you can begin the bath or shower with it on. Often once it is wet, he/she is glad to have it removed.

The shared shower: Mr. Trask was recently admitted to a care facility. Any attempts by staff to get him to shower or bathe met with fierce resistance. Instead of forcing him to bathe, the facility called his wife to find out how she had bathed him at home. She said that she had showered with him and that it had been enjoyable for them both. The wife was invited to come in and shower with her husband at the facility, with the staff assuring privacy. She was glad to be involved in his care and to be able to continue this part of their relationship.

There are an infinite number of ways to keep someone clean without a battle. However, many of the methods described are done outside of a shower or tub, without running water. This, of course, means that the hair also must be washed in creative ways.

Creative Hair Washing Techniques

Many persons with dementia resist and fear getting their hair washed. The reasons for this are varied. The most common way for caregivers to be trained to shower someone is to start at the top with the hair and work down, working from the "cleanest to the dirtiest" parts.

Caregiver Wisdom

It is not necessary to use a lot of shampoo to get the hair clean. Just a little dab works well and is easier to rinse out. Also, usually it isn't necessary to wash the hair twice. These shortcuts save time and energy and make hair washing better for the person and you.
Kathy House, CNA, Fairlawn Good Samaritan
Health Center, Gresham, OR

This can cause fearful, angry, and agitated behaviors. It can be overwhelming to have soapy water running into your eyes while you are cold, naked, and vulnerable. You have to wonder at the wisdom of teaching people to start the shower with the most distressing activity.

It's also helpful to think about why, when, and how to wash the hair.

- Why: The goal of hair washing is to clean the person's hair in pleasant, or at least tolerable, ways.
- When: Wash hair only when it is dirty if people don't enjoy it. Waiting until the end of the shower to wash the hair works best with most individuals. Often it is necessary to separate hair washing from the rest of the bath.
- How: Cover the person with dry towels or a bath blanket. Then try one of the following methods:

Wet washcloth method: Sometimes simply wetting and rinsing the hair using wet washcloths is useful. It is surprising how little water is required to adequately cleanse the hair. These techniques work well for washing the hair outside of the shower room also. For example, you could use the basin and washcloth method with the person fully clothed by protecting the clothes with plastic and a towel on the shoulders.

Beauty parlor sink method: Going to the beauty parlor has been a pleasant experience for many women. Continuing this activity as long as possible is certainly desirable for reasons of familiarity, enhancing the person's physical appearance, and socialization. You can use the sink in the beauty parlor when no one else is there. It's comfortable, convenient, and familiar to many.

In-bed inflatable basin method: Washing the hair in bed with a soft, plastic, inflatable basin with a drainage tube (Figure 4.2) can be very simple and soothing. Place the person's head in the opening, padded with washcloths to make it warmer and softer. Pour water from a pitcher onto the hair. Avoid drops on the face or in the ears as this can cause distress. A good time for this is early morning or after a nap.

Dry or no-rinse shampoo method: There are a number of products that allow you to wash hair without using water. Some are powderlike substances and some are a liquid you rub into the hair and towel dry off. If you are using a liquid, it is helpful to

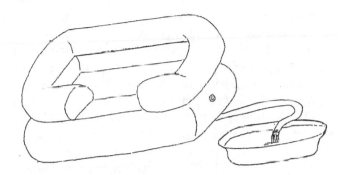

FIGURE 4.1 Inflatable basin.

warm it to body temperature before applying. Placing the bottle in the microwave or in warm water will do this. There is also a shower cap type of disposable product with no-rinse shampoo and conditioner that is heated in the microwave and placed on the person's head. The head is then massaged for 2–3 minutes and the cap removed. These no-rinse hair products can be useful as interim steps, but eventually the hair needs a more thorough rinsing.

Jelly-in-the-hair: When all your efforts fail you have to find a way to maintain both the person's appearance and right to say "no." Try finding a reason that the person will accept. One caregiver used "jelly-in-the-hair" as a last resort. Helen adamantly refused to let anyone wash her hair in spite of repeated attempts and approaches. She would bathe, but not let any water near her head. After many weeks of alternative methods, it was clear something else needed to be done. This facility subscribed to the philosophy of getting people to "yes" rather than forcing them to do something against their will. Georgia, a nursing assistant, had an idea. At breakfast, she "tripped" so the toast landed jelly side down on Helen's head. After apologizing and "cleaning" it off with a dry napkin, the woman could feel that her hair was still very sticky. Georgia asked her to come to the sink (hair washing sink) so she could try to get the jelly out, and was able to step-by-step add a little more water. Finally, she got Helen to agree to have her hair washed.

The Very Last Resort

Sometimes you can do your best, be creative, wait, try different approaches, and still fail to get the person to "yes." These instances will be very rare if you apply the principles of problem solving described here. There may be situations where there is a compelling health reason requiring that you go ahead with bathing in spite of protests. For example, when you are confronted with an incontinent person who has been sitting in a large, loose stool that is now getting all over, you need to do something quickly to prevent skin irritation and infection. Often in these situations, there may be some acute illness that is making the person uncomfortable and irritable. This needs further evaluation, but in the meantime you need to do something.

As a last resort, try the "good guy-bad guy" approach. Here you and another caregiver should carefully plan how you will bathe the person and have all supplies and equipment ready so it can be completed quickly and efficiently. One person talks to the person and loosely holds the hands to prevent him/her from striking you or the other staff member. This caregiver apologizes profusely to the person telling him/her that you understand that he/she doesn't like this and is angry or afraid. You reassure the individual that it will be over soon. The second person is efficiently but gently washing and cleaning the person. After the task is done it is important to debrief with the person, again apologizing. Doing something to soothe or bring pleasure to him/her (give a back rub or a cup of coffee) is a good thing to try, but often, he/she would prefer that you just get out of his/her sight!

Again, this approach should be reserved only for situations where there is a compelling health reason to bathe the individual against his/her will. Body odor without an underlying infection or skin breakdown is not a compelling reason. It has social implications, but not health ones. Family request is also not a compelling health reason. That requires education and partnering with the family to problem solve. Incontinence of both bowel and bladder can usually be cared for without the need for a full bath or shower. Therefore, in and of itself, incontinence is not a reason to "have to" put someone in a shower or tub to get them clean. Remember, when you proceed against a person's wishes he/she will feel attacked. We can't permit our routine care to support a practice where people feel they are being "attacked for their own good."

Finding Unique Solutions

There is not a set recipe for resolving concerns and dilemmas related to bathing. However, there are many common situations and suggested approaches that have been found to be useful. Some common situations include:

- does not want to bathe
- refuses to come into bathing area
- does not want to get undressed
- refuses to get into the tub/shower chair
- feels pain on movement
- skin is tender
- incontinence during bathing
- does not want feet washed
- does not want teeth brushed
- grabs or holds onto objects
- hollers or screams
- hits, kicks or slaps
- bites.

The chapter appendix contains tables that address each of these situations, the possible reasons for behaviors, suggested approaches and reasons why the approaches may be useful. Use the tables to individualize your approach and also stimulate your creativity and discover new solutions. Then share your ideas with your fellow workers.

Selecting solutions that fit individual needs and preferences can greatly increase the comfort of bathing for most persons with dementia. There are many different ways to maintain cleanliness. Set realistic goals for the bath and choose solutions based on your knowledge of the person. Observe the person's response and move on to the next step, evaluating the effectiveness of your solution.

Testing the Solutions

Did you meet your goal? Do additional changes need to be made? The best approach is to return to your original observations on the frequency and possible triggers of the behavioral symptom. Determine the level of improvement. You can record this on the Intervention Planning Table (see chapter appendix). For example, during your initial observations the person cried every time you to tried to wash between her toes with a washcloth. You hypothesized that this was due to pain since this person has arthritis. The solutions you chose were to first warn the person that you were going to wash between her toes, helping her get ready for the task. Then you used a Q-tip with warm water and soap to clean this area. She still cried, although her cries were not as loud or as long. She was quiet when you washed between her big toe and the second toe but her little toe seems particularly sensitive. You have made minimal progress towards your goal of meeting her need for a reduction in pain during the bath. You measure this lack of pain by a reduction in crying during feet washing. She is somewhat better. Again, you hypothesize about what is triggering the behavior. It could be that some areas of her feet are more sensitive than others and that you need a different approach.

Now you have to decide if there are other ways to meet your goal. Return to the list of possible solutions for feet washing. Which one is most likely to reduce her continued pain? You decide to separate feet washing from the bath and try soaking her feet in warm water and then washing them gently with a soft cloth. Again, you assess the effect of this new solution and find that she only cried once— when you touched the little toe on her right foot. This is good progress toward your goal. She is much better. You can decide to continue soaking her feet prior to washing them and each time assess the success or failure of this option.

SUMMARY

We have identified a three-step process that helps you develop a plan to address behavioral symptoms. This involves assessing and understanding the person and the behavior, and selecting, and then testing, solutions to meet individual needs. Your initial plan is just the beginning of the process that requires continual monitoring and readjustment. As cognitive or health status changes occur, you will also need to modify your plan to meet the changing needs of the person.

NOTE

The material in this chapter was adapted with permission from: Rader, J., & Barrick, A. L. (2000). Ways that work: Bathing without a battle, *Alzheimer's Care Quarterly, 1*(4), 35 49.

APPENDIX

- **Intervention Planning Table:** Use this form when trying out new solutions. It will help you and other caregivers know what new solutions have been tried, how they have worked, and ideas to try.

  - Photocopy it
  - Place it in the person's flowchart
  - Each time you bathe the person record observations of:

    - The behavior
    - The possible cause
    - The goal
    - The solution tried
    - The effectiveness of the solution
    - Any comments about why the solution helped or made things worse
    - Your plan for the next bath

- **Solution Tables:** These tables can be helpful in identifying different solutions to try when individualizing your approach. Once you have chosen a behavior, consult the appropriate table. Find the possible cause you have determined for the behavior, then select a solution to try. Add new solutions to the list as you discover them.

Today's Date ___ / ___ / ___

INTERVENTION PLANNING TABLE

Instructions: Record interventions and the results for each bath. Use Bathing Book to help with developing the plan.

Name: _____

Behavioral Symptom	Possible Cause	Goal	Solution	Effective-ness (see coding below*)	Comments (describe behavior)	Plan

*The intervention made the problem: 1 = Worse   2 = Somewhat worse   3 = No change   4 = Somewhat better   5 = Better

Comments: _____

_____

FIGURE 4.2   Intervention planning table.

TABLE 4.6 Person Doesn't Want to Bathe

Possible Reason	Action	Explanation
Personal		
Pain	Invite the person to the bath after pain meds have had a chance to alleviate person's discomfort.	Relief of pain associated with transfer, transport, and bath-related tasks may change how the person feels about the possibility of a bath
	Use a different method of transfer	Is less disruptive to person
Person has difficulty with transitions—leaving one location or activity for another	Take advantage of natural transition times. Invite the person into bathing area when walking by it and/or is already up and about	
Person needs other incentives for bathing	Offer a reward: Try a favorite activity or food	A treat makes bathing seem less unpleasant and can be motivating
Person may not be feeling up to it now	Try later	The initial reaction may be a passing sentiment. Acknowledging the person's feeling may affect how the person responds. Gives him/her some control
Person has difficulty with mobility	Use wheelchair or other device to help the person get to the shower	Walking to the bath may be very tiring/painful for some people
Interpersonal/Relationship		
Person may not understand that he/she needs a bath	Create a reason: Say it is time to freshen up for an activity, work or visitors; that his/her clothes look uncomfortable or need to be changed. Walk or talk with the person for a few minutes before inviting to bathe	Person may want to know why it is time to bathe. Builds trust prior to asking person to do something
Person has caregiver preferences	Delay until preferred caregiver is available. Try another caregiver, or invite a family member to help. If not usual caregiver or if a preference cannot be honored, talk to the person about that. Are there gender issues?	Person may prefer a different caregiver; or someone with whom he/she has a closer relationship Acknowledgement of preferences can positively affect a person's response to a less desirable situation
Person needs a quiet approach	Approach the person alone	A crowd of people may seem threatening

(continued)

TABLE 4.6 Person Doesn't Want to Bathe (*continued*)

Possible Reason	Action	Explanation
Physical Environment		
Room temperature or water temperature	Check room temperature before bringing person for bathing, check water temperature frequently	Older persons may be especially sensitive to temperature variations
Noise	Reduce amount of noise or conversation with anyone other than the person being bathed	Multiple sensory events can be disturbing to cognitively impaired person
Privacy	Keep person covered as much as possible. Bathe only one person at a time.	Feels safer and more respectful of privacy needs
Device used to transport persons is uncomfortable	Try different transportation method. Add cushions or other padding for comfort or positioning	Provides increased comfort and support for the person resulting in less resistance
Uncomfortable shower chair	Use an appropriately sized chair; and/or use water-resistant cushions; pad chair	Small individuals may not get adequate support in a large shower chair. Large persons may feel cramped. Pads provide cushioning and additional support
Organizational Environment		
Time of day	Determine if person prefers to be bathed at a particular time of day. Use information when setting up bath schedule.	Natural body rhythms vary among individuals. Accommodating these variations may change how a person reacts to the prospect of a bath
Mode of bathing	Determine whether person would prefer a tub, shower, or bed bath. If person is unable to respond, talk to other staff and/or family members. Try different ways of bathing	Accommodates person's preference. Also, gives a choice and a feeling of control

TABLE 4.7 Person Doesn't Want to Come to the Bathing Area

Possible Reason	Action	Explanation
Personal		
Doesn't want to bathe right now	Try later	Person may not be feeling up to it now
Fear	Approach person alone	A crowd of people may seem threatening
Control	Offer a reward. Try a favorite activity or food	A treat makes bathing seem less unpleasant and can provide motivation to bathe
	Invite the person for a walk without mentioning "bath"	Distracts person and avoids struggle
	Ask if he/she would prefer a tub, shower, or bed bath	Give person a choice and a feeling of control
Interpersonal/Relationship		
Doesn't recognize you	Try another caregiver, or invite a family member to help	Person may prefer a different caregiver or someone with whom he/she has a closer relationship
Doesn't trust you	Walk or talk with the person for a few minutes before inviting the person to bathe	Builds trust prior to asking the person to do something
Physical		
Unfamiliar environment	Assess if someone or something in the bathing area is contributing to the refusal	Aspects of the room, such as lighting, temperature, or another resident may provoke refusal
	Bathe in another location, such as in own room	Avoid transferring person to an unfamiliar or scary place. Person may be more comfortable in own room
Uncomfortable equipment	Try different transportation method, such as a wheelchair	Resident may want or need some assistance

TABLE 4.8 Person Doesn't Want to Get Undressed

Possible Reason	Action	Explanation
Personal		
Control	Have person choose clothes to be worn after the bath	Gives a sense of control over what is happening
	Create a reason: Say "You'll look nice in clean clothes" or "your clothes are dirty"	Gives a reason to undress
	Praise helping efforts	Encourages assistance
	Accept the refusal and offer to check back later	Gives a sense of control/autonomy
	Offer choices "Shall I undo your belt or do you want to?"	Allows some control over events
Fear	Reassure often	May feel attacked. Helps feel more secure
	Explain what you are doing in very simple words	May feel attacked. Helps understand
	Move slowly and gently, avoiding any "rushing" or fast movements	Going too quickly may frighten and confuse person
	Start by taking off shoes	Less threatening than taking upper body clothing off
Modesty	Undress from under a covering, such as wrapping a towel around the waist before removing pants	Maintains privacy
Cold	Keep person covered as often as possible with towels or with a blanket	May keep from feeling cold
Interpersonal/Relationship		
Doesn't understand your request	Try gesturing or physical guidance	May help understand
	Use distraction	May help gain cooperation if person can focus on something else
Doesn't recognize you as a caregiver	Introduce yourself and give time to understand	May help gain cooperation
Physical		
Room temperature is cool	Heat room prior to asking to undress	Helps keep the person comfortable
Organizational		
Different caregivers several times a week	Make permanent care assignments	Allows for the caregiver to get to know the person well and build the relationship

TABLE 4.9 Person Refuses to Get into Tub/Shower or Sit in Tub or on Shower Chair

Possible Reason	Action	Explanation
Personal		
Control	Have person test water temperature	Involves person in the activity; providing a sense of control over what is happening
	Praise helping efforts	Encourages assistance
	Bathe standing in shower using aqua socks or using pvc pipe walker or walking frame	Promotes safety and feeling of autonomy. Is more familiar way to shower
	Accept the refusal and offer to check back later	Provides sense of control and autonomy. Promotes relationship
Fear of falling	Reassure person that he/she won't fall ("We have you," "You'll be safe with me")	Person may be afraid of falling. Helps feel more secure
	Let person support self during transfer and seating using available handholds/bars	Person feels supported, in control during movements
	Get assistance if needed and appropriate	Additional support may be reassuring if person is afraid of falling
	Bathe the person standing in the tub and have person hold grab bars (maintain safety)	Avoids struggle. Helps feel more secure
	Call family to get history	May have negative fears/beliefs from past
Physical Environment		
Uncomfortable furnishings	Use chairlift or shower chair, if available	Person may have difficulties with limb movement and assistance makes person more comfortable
	Try a different type of bath	May be more comfortable
Bathroom looks unfamiliar, unfriendly	Create "friendlier" looking bathrooms	Person may be less fearful
	Verbally orient person to the room and equipment	Person may be less fearful
Interpersonal/Relationship Issues		
Doesn't understand your request	Apply gentle pressure behind knee with a chair or your hand to stimulate sitting	Physical cues may be more helpful than verbal ones for some persons
	Break down the task into simple, step-by-step movements; match communication level with ability	Entire action may be too complex for person to know what to do first
	Try a different kind of bath (e.g., in-room bath)	Reduces demands on person unable to understand what you are asking
Prefers a different caregiver	Try getting another person to do it	You may remind him/her of someone else

TABLE 4.10 If Person Feels Pain on Movement

Possible Reason	Action	Explanation
Personal		
Pain	Distract with conversation or food	Helps the person relax and may add something pleasant to the experience. Makes it an event rather than an unpleasant task
	When rolling over, roll the person onto the side that causes least discomfort	Reduces discomfort
Control	Have person hold bed rail and assist with turning	Gives the person a sense of control. Makes the move easier because person can assist
	Ask what will help and wait for a response if the person can talk	Can learn what person prefers. Helps feel connected to caregiver
Fear	Count with the person before moving	Helps the person prepare for move and give assistance rather than resistance. Replaces fear, avoids surprises, and distracts
	Reassure	Helps the person to feel more secure
	Use soothing tone	Helps to relax
	Move slowly	Gives the person time to adjust. Promotes a feeling of security
Organizational Environment		
	Get physical therapy consult to determine best method of transfer	Transfers are complex and need to be individualized for the safety and comfort of both the staff and person
	Use two to transfer	Can move the person more gently and give needed support. Reduces discomfort

TABLE 4.11 Skin Is Tender

Possible Reason	Action	Explanation
Personal		
Pain	Wash gently using a soft touch	Less friction reduces discomfort
	Use baby washcloths	They are softer than most washcloths
	Pat dry instead of rub	Avoids friction. Gentler on tender skin
	Start with the least sensitive area	Causes less distress
	Touch gently before beginning to wash	Helps the person adjust to touch
	Start with the least sensitive area	Causes less distress
	Use warmed wipe on rectum	These are softer than most washcloths
Control	Ask for feedback: "Does this feel OK?"	Lets the person know you care
Physical Environment		
Uncomfortable furnishings	Pad shower chair. Try a different kind of bath	May be more comfortable. Shower spray may cause discomfort
	Tell what you are going to do before doing it	Gives person a warning so will be prepared. Avoids surprises
Interpersonal/Relationship Issues		
Doesn't understand	Explain what you are doing	Helps feel understood

TABLE 4.12 Person Is Incontinent During Bath

Possible Reason	Action	Explanation
Personal		
Bath given at time of routine bowel movement or urination	Investigate bowel routine and schedule bath around it. Toilet first	Prevention
Physical movement stimulates elimination	Toilet first	Prevention
Physical Environment		
Shower chair stimulates bowel movement	Toilet first	Prevention is key
	Give a different type of bath	Prevention is the key
	Use a shower chair with a bucket	Prevention
	Put a chux pad on floor	Helps with cleanup. Maintains safety
Running water stimulates elimination	Run bathwater before person enters the room	Prevention is the key
	Toilet first	Prevention is key here

TABLE 4.13 Doesn't Want Feet Washed

Possible Reason	Action	Explanation
Personal		
Pain	Soak feet in a basin while sitting in shower chair	Feels good and loosens dirt
	Place moist cotton balls on toes to soak prior to washing	Helps soften dirt and dry skin for easier and less painful cleaning
	Use gloved fingers instead of a washcloth to wash feet	Can feel more like a massage. Easier to get to hard-to-reach places.
	Place feet on a dry towel and cover with another small towel and pat dry. Wash and dry between the toes with something thin and soft (e.g., dry washcloth, baby washcloth, cotton swab)	Less friction and joint pain. Allows for more gentle action than a washcloth in hard-to-reach places
Control	Ask for feedback. Have wash own feet if possible	Communicates respect
	Apologize at any sign of pain	Communicates respect
Physical Environment		
Uncomfortable furnishings	Support feet and legs with a stool covered with a towel	Helps with circulation and to feel more secure

TABLE 4.14 Person Doesn't Want Teeth Brushed

Reason	Action	Explanation
Personal		
Pain	Use a child's toothbrush	Smaller and softer and avoids pain
	Use child's toothpaste	Tastes sweet
Fear	Warn person of upcoming sensations and explain what you are doing	Avoids surprises and gives person time to prepare
	Do one step at a time	Decreases confusion as entire action may be too complex
	Distract with conversation about family, hobbies, food	Helps to distract person and may add some pleasure to the bathing experience
	Sing songs the person likes	Distracts person and helps relax
	Remain calm	Reassures person
	Reassure frequently	Promotes feeling of safety
Interpersonal/Relationship		
Trust	Apologize at any sign of pain	Validates the person and helps feel understood

TABLE 4.15 Person Grabs and Holds Onto Objects

Possible Reason	Action	Explanation
Personal/Interpersonal		
Pain	Support during transfers	Grabbing may reflect pain
	Try a different type bath	Avoids transfers or lifting that may cause pain
Does not understand	Give person something to hold such as a cloth, ball, figurine towel	Distracts person. Keeps hands occupied. Helps feel more secure
Fear	Have person hold grab-bars, tub, or seat	During transfer, person may grab because of fear of falling; helps feel more secure
	Provide more support, both verbal and physical (e.g., another caregiver) during transfers. Involve PT/OT to determine best method for transfer	Grabbing may reflect the person's fear and need for security
	Try a different kind of bath (e.g., in-room bath, or shower instead of a tub bath)	Avoids transfers or lifting which may have made the person fearful
Control	Consider letting person hold onto object you are trying to remove. Be flexible and stay calm.	It is okay for person to hold onto clothing, towels, or other personal items
	Have the person help (e.g., wash face).	Keeps hands occupied. May give person a sense of control
Doesn't want to bathe	Come back another time	May not feel good; respects choice
Interpersonal/Relationship		
Doesn't understand what is happening	Explain each step. Match communication to abilities	Improves understanding
Your pacing varies from person to person	Pace your approach to his/her pace	Moving too fast can overwhelm the person
Physical Environment		
Ill-fitting shower chair creates discomfort	Purchase a short chair for a small person, or put a stool under the person's feet	Helps person feel more supported and secure

TABLE 4.16 Person Hollers or Screams

Possible Reason	Action	Explanation
Personal		
Pain	Stop what you are doing and assess what may be causing the pain or discomfort	Helps alleviate source of pain
	Apologize	Helps person feel understood
	Try a different type of bath	A bed bath may be less painful
	Use a very gentle touch	Skin may be very sensitive
	Try a baby washcloth	Softer and causes less pain
Fear	Warn the person of upcoming sensations by gently touching area and telling person what you are going to do	Eliminates frightening surprises
	Reduce water pressure or use a different way to rinse person	Water spray can frighten person
	Try music. Have the person or family choose a favorite song or tape to play.	Can be soothing and help the person relax
	Sing with the person	Can be soothing and distracting
	Reduce the number of people present	"Strangers" may pose a threat
	Converse with the person	Helps relax and distract. May stop yelling to answer
Control	Give choices	Gives person a sense of control
	Converse with the person about favorite topics	Helps feel understood, valued
Cold	Put warm water on washcloth	Reduces discomfort of cold cloth
Interpersonal/Relationship		
Doesn't feel understood	Respond with concern each time the person hollers	Helps person feel understood and builds relationship
Physical Environment		
Uncomfortable equipment	Adapt equipment to the person	Equipment may be painful and causing yelling
Noisy environment	Try bathing in a quieter environment	Noise may be upsetting

TABLE 4.17 Person Hits, Kicks, or Slaps During Bath

Possible Reason	Action	Explanation
Personal		
Desire for control	Encourage person to help, if possible, with the bath. Often this works well when washing the genital/rectal areas or painful areas.	Since person may be feeling assaulted, getting person involved allows him/her a feeling of control over what is happening. More dignified
	Say firmly that the behavior is unacceptable, such as "that hurts" or "stop kicking"	Lets person know the behavior is not okay and should stop
	Try the good-guy/bad-guy approach: Assign one person to bathe and another to hold the person's hands gently while talking with the person.	This methods gets a very unpleasant task done quickly and protects caregivers from harm. Should be used only as a last resort
	Give choices, ask permission	Helps person feel more control
Pain	Stop what you are doing.	Gives opportunity to assess what may be causing the aggression.
	Apologize	Helps person feel more understood
	Explore giving pain medication prior to bathing	Elders have many potential sources of pain related to bathing. Agitation and aggression are often precipitated by pain.
Fear	Give person something to hold such as cloth, soap, or someone's hands. Use interesting objects (color and texture, side of shower, chair, towel)	Gives person's hands something else to do. Distracts
	Call person's name firmly and directly, without yelling	Person will stop and listen
	Reassure that you're not trying to hurt him/her	Helps alleviate fear
	Learn defensive self-protection techniques such as blocking blows	Protect yourself from harm
Interpersonal/Relationship		
Doesn't understand what is happening	Slow down, or stop: Ask what is wrong	Lets person know you see him/her as a person, not a task to be done
	Apologize repeatedly and sincerely. Attempt to remedy complaints	Respects person. Helps feel understood.
Physical Environment		
Uncomfortable surrounding	Check comfort of seating device, temperature of water and room noise level	Problems in these areas can cause aggression
Organizational Environment		
No flexibility in time or form of bathing	Slow down, stop, ask what is wrong, make more comfortable. Discuss with RN or other staff the need for flexibility in the future	Person will feel respected. Organization will be more responsive.

TABLE 4.18 Person Bites

Possible Reason	Action	Explanation
Personal		
Fear	Reassure	Decreases anxiety
	Engage person in singing or humming	Keeps person's mouth busy with other activity; distracts
Pain	Explore giving pain meds before you start	Pain is often related to aggression
Hunger	Give person gum to chew, or other item such as cookies or beverage (water)	Keeps person's mouth busy with other activity. Helps alleviate hunger
	Bathe after eating	Prevention is the key
Interpersonal/Relationship		
Doesn't understand/can't inhibit behavior	Beware of mouth if person has a history of biting	Prevent self from getting hurt
	Offer alternatives during bite like gum, candy	Keeps person's mouth busy
	Identify mildly agitated behaviors that occur before biting and take action or back off at that point	Person may bite when very agitated. Try to prevent person from reaching that point
	If has dentures, don't put them in until after bath, unless person objects	Won't hurt as much!

Part II

Special Concerns

CHAPTER 5

Preserving Abilities:
Finding the Best Level of Assistance

Carla Gene Rapp, Valorie Shue,
and Cornelia Beck

SELECTING THE BEST LEVEL OF ASSISTANCE FOR ACTIVITIES OF DAILY LIVING

When we get dressed in the morning, it is usually a practical activity to get covered, warm, and ready for the day—an activity we do without much thought. For example, we do not think about how we fasten buttons. We may be more conscious of dressing and taking pleasure in it if we are going somewhere special, but generally, dressing is just a task to be done. The same is true for bathing, a task necessary to keep skin clean and free from odor, dirt, and germs, but one we rarely think much about. Dressing and bathing are activities that are commonly done sequentially. Bathing starts with undressing and ends with dressing. Although dressing and bathing are often simple and unconscious activities for people without cognitive or physical limitations, they can be very frustrating experiences for the caregiver and the person with dementia for numerous reasons, including physical limitations, pain, or cognitive changes.

Most persons with dementia have disabilities in one or more of four specific areas: 1) attention, 2) language (seen as the inability to follow one-step commands), 3) sequencing, and 4) judgment. Each person's individual disabilities can guide you, the caregiver, in deciding how much help the person needs. The amount of help is called the "level of assistance." Table 5.1 contains definitions and suggestions for when to use each level of assistance.

Each level of assistance has specific strategies associated with it. Because dementia affects persons in differ-

ent ways over time, you need to individualize the strategies to each person's needs. With the right prompts and assistance, persons can use preserved skills and function more independently. When you provide too much (or the wrong kind of) assistance, excess disability occurs. A person with excess disability looks more impaired than he or she actually is. We often do not know how much ADL dependence is related to actual physical or cognitive impairment or caused by improper medications, problems in the physical environment, or caregiver beliefs and behaviors (all potential factors in creating excess disability). However, no matter the cause, using strategies to maximize the person's strengths and increase feelings of success can reduce excess disability.

Caregiver Wisdom

Your approach has to match the person's needs and abilities. You need more than one trick up your sleeve. Plus, how you present yourself when you enter the room makes a difference.
Janine Nelson, CNA, CMA, Providence Benedictine Nursing Center, Mt. Angel, OR

Imagine that this is the first day that you are providing care to Mrs. J., a 78-year-old woman with dementia. Other caregivers have talked about their experiences helping Mrs. J. get bathed and dressed, saying that she "never helps," that you "need to do everything for her," and that she "always complains about what she is wear-

TABLE 5.1 Levels of Assistance and When to Use Them

Level of Assistance	Definition	When to Use
ENVIRONMENTAL MODIFICATION:	Altering the environment to cue or encourage an action—for example, closing the door to reduce distractions or laying clothes out in the correct order.	Helps the person who has problems putting things in order, paying attention, and making good decisions. Compensates for these problems by controlling what is around the person.
VERBAL PROMPT:	Asking the person to begin the action or talking him or her through the task.	Helps the person who has trouble starting or following through on a task. When the person cannot tell left from right, give verbal prompts, saying "this," "that," and "the other," instead of "right" or "left." The prompts help the person who has trouble both understanding when someone speaks to him/her and paying attention. Repeat your prompts if a person processes slowly. Use this strategy with a person who does not understand words, but always with a strategy that does not require verbal understanding.
MODELING/GESTURING:	Demonstrating or "acting out" the task for the person to imitate or using gestures to start or guide the person through the task.	Helps the person who has trouble speaking or understanding words and paying attention, but can imitate actions. Sometimes modeling/gesturing works better if you also use words (verbal prompts).
PHYSICAL PROMPT:	Touching the person to attract his or her attention or to indicate which part of the body to move.	Helps the person who can both start and continue a task but has problems understanding words. These prompts refocus the person's attention or help direct his or her actions. Use physical prompts with verbal prompts to help the person better understand what you want him or her to do.
PHYSICAL GUIDANCE:	Guiding the person through the task by assisting him or her to make the body movements necessary to complete the task. When using physical guidance, start the activity for the person, then allow him or her to complete the activity independently.	Helps the person who cannot start or imitate an action, but can carry through once you start the step. This person usually has problems understanding words as well. Guide the person's movements when giving help with a task. Do movements "with" not "for" the person.
OCCASIONAL PHYSICAL GUIDANCE:	Providing minimal physical guidance only when the person gets distracted or is not responding. The person who requires occasional guidance can start the activity, but at times requires your assistance to restart or redirect an action.	Helps the person who can start but cannot continue an activity and has trouble understanding words. Only give physical guidance when the person stops responding.
COMPLETE PHYSICAL GUIDANCE:	Performing all necessary body movements while guiding the person through the steps of a task.	Helps the person who cannot start, imitate, or continue an action. The person usually has problems speaking or understanding words as well.

ing." Upon entering her room, you find her sitting on the side of the bed, trying to eat her breakfast. You notice that her food has not been cut, nor have the sealed containers been opened. You ask if she needs help cutting her food and opening the containers. She replies that she does, and you help. When you finish, she starts eating again.

Based on your first meeting with her, would you expect that you should have to completely bathe and dress Mrs. J.? What leads you to this conclusion? What specific activities would you do when helping Mrs. J. with her bathing and dressing? This chapter will describe a decision-making process that you can use to identify what level of assistance and what specific strategies will enable a person with dementia to do as much as possible without help.

Determining the Right Level of Assistance

To maximize the person's abilities, you must first find out how much help (level of assistance) a person needs. The decision-making process of choosing the appropriate level of assistance is fairly simple and will be presented both in the text that follows and in Table 5.2.

The process involves asking a series of questions.

Question 1. **Can the person sequence and make good judgments?** Difficulty sequencing means the person does a task with steps in the wrong order (i.e., picks up washcloth, wipes face with it, attempts to apply soap, wets washcloth, puts cloth down). Impaired judgment means the person makes unsuitable decisions (does not try to stay clean or have a neat appearance; wears underclothes on top of shirt or pants). When the person has trouble sequencing or making good judgments, he or she will need at least ENVIRONMENTAL MODIFICATION. Regardless of your answer here, go to Question 2 (See Table 5.2).

Question 2. **Can you gain the person's attention easily?** If you can, the person will notice you when you enter the room or when you speak in a normal tone of voice. If you cannot easily gain the person's attention, the person will ignore you, or you will need to touch the person or speak loudly to get the person's attention. If you cannot gain attention easily, go to Question 3. If you can gain attention easily, then use your answer from Question 1 (whether or not the person can sequence and make good judgments):

a. If so, the person needs no assistance.
b. If not, the person needs ENVIRONMENTAL MODIFICATION.

Question 3. **Can the person maintain attention and understand words?** If yes, the correct level of assistance is ENVIRONMENTAL MODIFICATION. However, if the person is able to pay attention for only short periods and ignores people, objects, and sounds, then go to Question 4.

Question 4. **Can the person follow one-step commands?** Ask the person to do a simple task that he/she should be able to do (i.e., touch your nose, close your eyes). If he/she can, use VERBAL PROMPT. If he/she cannot, go to Question 5.

Question 5. **Can the person start an activity?** Because the person cannot follow one-step commands, spoken instructions alone will fail. Try nonverbal and physical methods of communication. To find out if the person can start a task, see if the person can use a common object correctly (lift cup to mouth) when you put the item in front of (or hand it to) him or her. If the person can start a task, go to Question 5A. If the person cannot start a task, go to Question 6.

Question 5A. To Question 5, you answered that the person could start a task. Now ask: **Can the person continue that task?** Watch the person while he/she does the task. (Place the cup in front of the person, touch his or her hand, and see if he/she picks up the cup, starts drinking from it, and continues until satisfied.) If the person can both start and continue a task, use a PHYSICAL PROMPT since the person has a hard time understanding words. If the person can start a task but forgets to continue a task, he/she will need OCCASIONAL PHYSICAL GUIDANCE whenever he/she stops doing the task.

Question 6. **Can the person imitate or do a movement** (clap hands, touch chin)? Usually if the person cannot start a task, he/she cannot imitate. If the person can imitate, the person needs the level of assistance called MODELING/GESTURING. If the person cannot imitate, ask Question 7.

Question 7. **Can the person continue an activity?** To do this, start a task and see if the person can complete it. (Place comb in hand and lift hand with comb to head. See if he/she then combs hair.) When the person can continue a task, he/she will need PHYSICAL GUIDANCE to start the task, but

TABLE 5.2 Choosing the Correct Level of Assistance

Question	Answer	Caregiver Response
Question 1. Can the person sequence or made good judgments?	• Yes • No	Ask Question 2 Provide at least ENVIRONMENTAL MODIFICA-TION and ask Question 2
Question 2. Can you gain the person's attention easily, and can the person sequence and make good judgments?	• Yes and a. Person *can* sequence and make good judgments b. Person *cannot* sequence or make good judgments • No	Provide no assistance Provide ENVIRONMENTAL MODIFICATION Ask Question 3
Question 3. Can the person maintain attention and understand spoken words?	• Yes • No	Provide ENVIRONMENTAL MODIFICATION Ask Question 4
Question 4. Can the person follow one-step commands?	• Yes • No	Provide VERBAL PROMPT Ask Question 5
Question 5. Can the person start a task?	• Yes • No	Ask Question 5A Ask Question 6
Question 5A. Can the person continue a task?	• Yes • No	Provide PHYSICAL PROMPT Provide OCCASIONAL PHYSICAL GUIDANCE
Question 6. Can the person imitate?	• Yes • No	Provide MODELING/GESTURING Ask Question 7
Question 7. Can the person continue a task?	• Yes • No	Provide PHYSICAL GUIDANCE Provide COMPLETE PHYSICAL GUIDANCE

probably can follow through without help. However, if the person cannot continue a task, he/she will need COMPLETE PHYSICAL GUIDANCE to both start and finish the task.

Strategies to Match the Level of Assistance

At this point, you have figured out what level of assistance the person needs. Each level of assistance has different strategies that let you give the right amount of help. Usually, you will use all of the strategies for the chosen level of assistance. In addition, you may use some of the strategies from levels that provide less help. Only in rare cases will you use strategies that give more help. Refer to Table 5.3 for a listing of the specific strategies suggested for each level of assistance, as well as for tips on how and when to use them.

Caregiver Wisdom

I try to set it up so it is easy for them. As a person begins to lose skills as part of the dementia, you have to continually adjust. You want to maintain the person's abilities, but if he/she becomes too frustrated, you want to offer assistance in a way that allows him/her to maintain dignity.

Beth Parker, Marian Estates, Sublimity, OR

Standard Strategies

Standard strategies are used with everyone who needs assistance. Table 5.4 presents the standard strategies and tips on how and when to use them.

The first two strategies (one-step commands and verbal praise) clearly apply when the person can understand words; however, even when the person generally does not understand words, this strategy creates a calm and respectful atmosphere. Also, there is a chance that the person will understand the meaning or intent (if not the words). The next two standard strategies require individualization (choosing appropriate/desired reinforcers and identifying the best way to structure the activity), but should apply to anyone with dementia. The final strategy (anticipating the need for help) requires that you know the correct level of assistance

strategies to use. When you know the kind and amount of help the person needs, and at what point the person needs that help, you are more likely to be able to assist in a manner that will allow maximum ADL independence. Overall, the standard strategies are simply a way to make the level of assistance strategies work better.

Case Study

Mr. B., an 84-year-old white male, has dementia, hypertension, and Parkinson's disease. You notice that during morning care he often does things in the wrong order (tries to wash with a washcloth that is neither wet, nor has soap on it) and insists on wearing a short sleeve shirt without a jacket, no matter how cold the weather. To get Mr. B.'s attention, you have to be right in front of him, and touch him so he will look at you. Even if you can gain his attention, it usually wanders after a minute or two (and usually he walks away as well). He rarely speaks and appears to understand what you say to him only part of the time. Mr. B. rarely starts a task without help, but he will imitate the movements that you make (miming picking up a pair of pants from the bed).

As Mr. B.'s caregiver you can use the decision-making process described in this chapter to help you decide what level of assistance Mr. B. needs, and then to select strategies to use when caring for him. Begin with Table 5.2, and ask the questions there.

Question 1. **Can the person sequence or make good judgments?** No, Mr. B. cannot sequence or make good judgment.

Question 2. **Can you gain the person's attention easily, and can the person sequence and make good judgments?** No, it is very hard to gain Mr. B.'s attention.

Question 3. **Can the person maintain attention and understand spoken words?** No, once gained, Mr. B.'s attention wanders easily, and he has difficulty understanding spoken words.

Question 4. **Can the person follow one-step commands?** No, Mr. B. does not understand words and therefore cannot follow one-step commands.

Question 5. **Can the person start a task?** No, Mr. B. rarely starts a task alone.

TABLE 5.3 Levels of Assistance and Suggested Strategies: How and When to Use Them

Specific Strategy	How and When to Use
	ENVIRONMENTAL MODIFICATION
Use a solid color background that is dark to contrast dressing or bathing items.	Use a dark colored bedspread as a background when putting out clothes to use in dressing. This strategy helps the person who cannot tell shades, colors, or patterns apart.
Arrange items in the position and order in which the person will use them.	Arrange Mr. D.'s clothes facedown in a pile on the bed from bottom to top in this order: belt, shirt, undershirt, pants, socks, and underwear. Thus, the first item Mr. D. will put on is on the top of the pile, and the last item is on the bottom. This strategy helps the person with problems sequencing.
Hand items in the correct position.	Hand Mr. G. his brush with the handle facing him so that when he takes it, he can start brushing his hair without having to turn it around first. This strategy also works well with putting items in the right order and position.
Place item(s) beside the part of the body that the person will use to finish the task.	Cue Mrs. W. to put on her shoes by placing each shoe by the correct foot. For this strategy to work, the person must be able to see the item when you place it by the part of the body and move well enough to start the task.
Reduce number of options available (let person choose from only two options).	Allow Mrs. K. some control when putting on her lipstick. Let her choose between one red and one pink instead of offering her all 10 lipsticks out of her drawer. This strategy helps when the person has poor judgment or wants control (especially when the person will complain or change clothes if he/she dislikes the clothes you have chosen, or will refuse to use items that you offer).
	VERBAL PROMPT
Introduce ADL items one at a time.	Say the name of each item (i.e., washcloth, soap, and towel) as Mr. P. picks it up or as you hand each item to him. Saying the name of each item may help him correctly recognize it.
Provide brief, simple verbal directions.	Use this strategy by saying, "Mrs. C., pick up the shirt. Put your arm in the sleeve. Pull the shirt around your back. Put your other arm in the other sleeve. Pull the front closed. Fasten the buttons." The person may need verbal prompts every so often or the whole time.
Repeat your verbal prompt.	Some people can respond to verbal prompts, but may need extra time to process (i.e., time for their brain to figure what their body is supposed to do). To increase the amount of processing time, count to 10 before repeating the prompt.

(continued)

TABLE 5.3 Levels of Assistance and Suggested Strategies: How and When to Use Them *(continued)*

Specific Strategy	How and When to Use
	MODELING/GESTURING
Show the person what to do (point to the item that the person will use, or show the person how to do a step of dressing/bathing by making the right motion for that step yourself).	Point to Mr. S.'s toothbrush as a signal for him to pick up the brush. Then act out placing the brush under running water.
	PHYSICAL PROMPT
Use physical touch to show the person which part of the body to use.	Touch Mrs. W.'s left leg if you want her to lift it. To use both verbal and physical prompts, touch the leg while saying, "Lift this leg." This strategy also helps get the person's attention.
	PHYSICAL GUIDANCE
Use physical guidance to start the person's movement, then allow the person to complete the action without help.	Place the washcloth in Mr. Z.'s hand, guide his hand to the water to get the washcloth wet, and guide the washcloth to a soaped area of skin. Mr. Z. then rinses off the soap.
	OCCASIONAL PHYSICAL GUIDANCE
Provide minimal physical guidance to restart a task only until the person resumes the task without help.	When Mrs. Y. stops washing her arm, move Mrs. Y.'s hand in a washing motion until she resumes washing on her own.
	COMPLETE PHYSICAL GUIDANCE
Perform all body movements while guiding the person through the steps of a task.	Lift Mr. K.'s arm and guide it through the sleeve of his shirt, then lift the other arm and guide it through the other sleeve. Guide his hands to pull the shirt closed in the front and into the correct position.
Use reverse chaining (graduated physical guidance) by allowing the person to finish the step and decrease help as the person is able to do more.	On day one, assist Mrs. N. as outlined above. On day two, provide complete physical guidance until it is time to pull the shirt into the right position. At this point, stop helping to see if Mrs. N. will complete the task. Continue doing less and less physical guidance as Mrs. N. does more without help. This strategy works best when the person can finish a task, but can't start it.

TABLE 5.4 Standard Strategies: How and When to Use Them

Strategy	How and When to Use
One-Step Commands	• Speak simple sentences with as few words as possible. • Tell Mrs. D. each step to perform. "Unbutton your pants." "Unzip your pants." "Pull down your pants." "Sit." • If the person does not understand words, you cannot depend on these commands to work, but they may still be helpful. One-step commands may not work when used alone, but when used with other strategies, one-step commands may increase the person's independence. • Caregivers tend to ask questions and give "nonchoice" choices instead of simply making a statement. For example, caregivers ask, "Would you like to get up?" instead of stating, "I'm here to help you get up now."
Verbal Praise	• Use after completion of each step and after completing the entire task of dressing/bathing. • Say, "Mrs. S., you are doing a great job getting those knots out of your hair." "You look nice. . . you did a great job combing your hair this morning." • Use this strategy with almost everyone except for persons who cannot understand any words or do not respond to this type of support. When it is unclear if the person can understand words, use this strategy just in case the person understands the praise. • Use as many rewards as possible to encourage the person to take part in the activity of daily living.
Specific Reinforcement	• Find out what the person likes then use these as specific reinforcers. For example: knowing how much Mr. T. loves coffee, allow Mr. T. to have an extra cup of coffee when he shaves himself with as little help as possible. • Other examples of reinforcers include candy (may need to use sugar-free), reading a favorite magazine, or going for a walk.
Consistent Activity Structuring	• Every time, begin the ADL activity with a specified body part, then proceed with the specified body parts in the order that these steps are to be completed.
Anticipate the Need for Help	• This strategy works with the person who is unaware of his or her need for help or is unwilling or unable to ask for help. • For example, since you know that Mrs. B. cannot touch her toes, you will put the socks on her feet and pull them up to the point on her leg that she can reach to complete the step. • You may want to wait a period of time (count to 10) before giving help. This gives the person a chance to try to do the task before you help.

Question 6 **Can the person imitate?** Yes, Mr. B. can imitate an action. You now know the level of assistance that Mr. B. needs: MODELING/GESTURING.

Next, you will determine which of the specific strategies (from Tables 5.3 and 5.4, or the "prescription" form [see chapter appendix]) you should use. When selecting strategies, begin with the strategies (Table 5.3) for the level of assistance you determined in the decision-making process as demonstrated above. Mr. B.'s required level of assistance is MODELING/GESTURING, so you will use the strategy for this level (Table 5.3): Use modeling/gesturing to show Mr. B. what to do.

Then, you will consider the remaining level of assistance strategies:

ENVIRONMENTAL MODIFICATION: Hand items in the correct position. Select this strategy, since his Parkinson's causes a tremor that makes it hard for him to pick up items.

VERBAL PROMPT: Give verbal directions during bathing or dressing. Use this strategy in case he *does* understand the words.

PHYSICAL PROMPT: Use touch to show him which part of his body you want him to use. Choose this strategy to help Mr. B. focus on the task.

PHYSICAL GUIDANCE: No applicable strategies.

OCCASIONAL PHYSICAL GUIDANCE: No applicable strategies.

COMPLETE PHYSICAL GUIDANCE: No applicable strategies.

Next, review the standard strategies (Table 5.4). Expect to use all five of these, and be sure to find a specific reinforcer to strengthen the desired behaviors. Mr. B. will benefit from all of these strategies.

- Use one-step commands. Keep sentences simple: use one or two words if possible.
- Praise Mr. B. after he finishes each step and when he has completely bathed or dressed.
- Mr. B. loves ice cream. Give him a bowl as a reward after he completes the task.

- For dressing, begin with his *upper body*, then go to his *lower body*.
- Anticipate his need for help.

As time passes, Mr. B.'s condition may change, and you will need to use this process again to identify other strategies. By using these strategies when caring for Mr. B., we hope he will become more active in his care and more independent in bathing and dressing.

Conclusion

By using the decision-making process presented in this chapter, you can increase the ADL independence of persons with dementia. Consider each person's specific strengths and weaknesses. No strategy will work with every person, and the person's responses will vary from day-to-day. This makes working with the person a daily challenge. However, the decision-making process described in this chapter is one way to improve the quality of life and care of these persons. The process works equally well in acute-care hospitals, private homes, or nursing homes. Through use of these strategies, persons with dementia will be able to perform their activities of daily living as much as possible without help.

APPENDIX

Individualized ADL "Prescription" Form

Use the "prescription" form to determine specific strategies to use when assisting persons with dementia during ADL care. Fill in the specific information, identifying the person and their location. Circle or highlight each of the level of assistance and standard strategies that should be used with the person, being sure to fill in all of the blanks, where applicable. Other modifications to the strategies can also be written on this form. The form should then be kept somewhere that is accessible to anyone who will be assisting the person with his or her ADLs.

Individualized ADL "Prescription" Form

Person _____   Location _____

Level of Assistance Strategies

*ENVIRONMENTAL MODIFICATION:
Use a solid color background that is dark to contrast dressing or bathing item.
Arrange items in the position and order in which the person will use them.
Place item(s) beside the part of the body that the person will use to finish the task.
Hand items in the correct position.
Reduce number of options available (let the person choose from only two options).

*VERBAL PROMPT:
Introduce ADL items one at a time.
Provide brief, simple verbal directions.
Repeat your verbal prompt.

*MODELING/GESTURING:
Show the person what to do (point to the item that the person will use, or show the person how to do a step of dressing/bathing by making the right motion for that step yourself).

*PHYSICAL PROMPT:
Use physical touch to show the person which part of the body to use.

*PHYSICAL GUIDANCE:
Use physical guidance to start the person's movement, then allow the person to complete the action without help.

*OCCASIONAL PHYSICAL GUIDANCE:
Provide minimal physical guidance to restart a task only until the person resumes the task without help.

*COMPLETE PHYSICAL GUIDANCE:
Perform all body movements while guiding the person through the steps of a task.
Use reverse chaining (graduated physical guidance) by allowing the person to finish the step and decrease help as the person is able to do more.

Standard Strategies

Use one-step commands. Speak simple sentences with as few words as possible.

Give verbal praise. Use after completion of each step and after completing the entire task of dressing/bathing.

Offer specific reinforcement _____.

At each time that dressing/bathing is done, begin activity with _____
(specify body part), then proceed with _____
(specify body part(s) and/or order in which steps are to be completed).

Anticipate the need for help.

CHAPTER 6

Managing Pain

Karen Amann Talerico and Lois L. Miller

Pain has been identified as a cause of behavioral symptoms that leads to battles during bathing. Bathing provides multiple opportunities for pain stimulation due to transfers, movement of arms and legs, and touching or washing of body surfaces. However, the person with dementia is often unable to clearly communicate his or her pain or ask for relief. Most people with dementia will never have the ability to say, "I'd like my pain medication about an hour before I get my bath this morning." They may be left with only nonverbal ways to communicate discomfort, ways that have often been thought of as resistive or disruptive by caregivers. Such behaviors include pushing the caregiver away, hitting, or yelling. These behaviors become understandable as the person's response to protect himself/herself from pain, if you are able to understand that pain may be causing them.

Older people are more likely to suffer from arthritis, bone and joint disorders, back problems, and many other chronic conditions that are painful. Table 6.1 lists disorders that frequently lead to chronic pain in nursing home residents, with arthritis and osteoporosis being two of the most common. Untreated chronic pain has been associated with poor quality of life, depression, poor cognitive function, decreased socialization, sleep disturbances, and impaired walking. While most studies have been done with older adults in long-term care settings, there is no reason to think that pain issues are different for older adults who live in the community.

Even when pain is reported by older adults, most studies have identified an alarming trend towards leaving pain untreated in as many as 85% of older adults with identified pain and/or pain-causing diagnoses (Ferrell,

Ferrell, & Osterweil, 1990). Health care professionals have been found to underestimate the presence and severity of pain by as much as 50%–80%. Older adults with dementia are often given less analgesics than cognitively intact older adults, even with the same pain-causing conditions (Horgas & Tsai, 1998; Kaasalainen et al., 1998). Communication impairment has been identified as a major contributing factor to the underassessment and treatment of pain in advanced dementia.

Undertreatment of pain is also often due to opiophobia, the fear of getting someone addicted to opiate drugs. These fears are generally unfounded, and should only be given serious consideration in someone who has a previous history of addictive behavior. Even if someone has a history of addiction, they may need opioid medications to adequately treat pain. Luckily there is much that can be done about pain, once it is recognized.

TABLE 6.1   Frequent Causes of Pain and Discomfort in Older Adults

Acute injuries
Arthritis
Back pain
Cancer
Constipation
Contractures (frozen joints)
Dental problems
Gastrointestinal (stomach) disorders
Neuropathies (nerve pain)—diabetic, alcoholic, or postherpetic (after shingles)
Osteoporosis
Old fracture or injury sites
Pressure ulcers
Urinary tract problems, such as infection or spasms

Pain Assessment Tailored to Persons With Dementia

What can you do to improve the recognition and treatment of pain? The first step is to assess whether pain is in fact causing your bathing battle. Because pain is so common in older persons, and because many persons with dementia will not self-report pain or discomfort, all persons should be assessed for pain. Persons with dementia usually have very unique expressions of pain, and the individual approach recommended in this book is especially needed when it comes to pain assessment. One woman's unique pain expression was holding her hand to her forehead whenever she had discomfort. Her husband communicated this to the nursing staff, as it had been her lifelong pattern. This allowed her caregivers to know that when she held her hand to her forehead that they should do something to help relieve her discomfort. Some persons with dementia who are experiencing pain may become withdrawn and less willing to get out of bed, others yell and scream, some will moan, some increase the amount of pacing, while others may actually laugh. A comprehensive assessment should include all of the following areas.

Information on Painful Medical Conditions

One of the most important things is to obtain thorough information about the person's past and current medical problems that could be causing pain, such as arthritis, osteoporosis, old healed fractures, back pain, contractures, and cancer (Table 6.1). These sources of pain are not likely to go away as a person's dementia worsens, yet pain becomes more difficult to express verbally for the person with dementia. There is no solid evidence to suggest that people with dementia feel pain any differently than you or I do. It is also important to know how the person managed pain in the past, what treatments were effective, especially use of medications. Families can be important allies and sources of information in this process. This information can then be used to develop an individualized pain treatment plan for the person.

Direct Questioning

Persons with dementia who have a potentially painful condition should be asked directly if they are experienc-

ing pain. Start with the question, "Are you uncomfortable now?" Many confused persons can answer this simple question. It is important to know the amount of pain a person is experiencing so that treatment effectiveness can be assessed. Therefore, it is preferable to use a pain intensity rating scale, if possible. A number of rating scales are available such as the Present Pain Intensity Scale from the McGill Pain Questionnaire (Table 6.2 and chapter appendix). Studies have shown that older adults often have the ability to use at least one type of pain rating scale, even those with dementia, and that they prefer to use a scale with word descriptors rather than a scale with only numbers (Ferrell, Ferrell, & Rivera, 1995). It is important to find a scale that works best for each individual, rather than using one scale that may only work for some people. You may have to use a particular scale several times before the person is able to use it appropriately. It is also important to use this scale, which works for the person consistently over time to evaluate the course of the pain and its response to your treatment plan. The goal of successful pain treatment is to ensure that the pain intensity rating is below 4 on a 0–10 scale or below 3 (distressing) on a 0–5 scale. It may not always be possible to get chronic pain down to a zero on the rating scale.

Pain at the Moment

The person with dementia may not be able to recall pain during a previous time period, such as yesterday or even an hour ago, because of memory loss. Thus, you should monitor pain at the moment, as well as over time. You will then have information about pain relief and how effective treatments are for the person. Pain assessments should include a pain description, observation of nonverbal pain behaviors, alleviating or worsening factors, AND the effect of pain on the person's

TABLE 6.2 Present Pain Intensity from the McGill Pain Questionnaire (Melzack, 1975)

0	No pain
1	Mild
2	Discomforting
3	Distressing
4	Horrible
5	Excruciating

Reprinted by permission of the author, Ronald Melzack, PhD.

functional status (how much they walk and take care of themselves).

Pain Descriptors

It is important to use a variety of terms to describe pain to find one that is comfortable FOR THAT PERSON. Some older adults may say they have no pain, but then go on to talk about their discomfort, an aching or burning feeling, or that they are uncomfortable. Ask about the part of the body that you know has been painful in the past. For example, the person might respond negatively to the question, "Are you having any pain?" but respond positively to the question, "Is your back hurting?" or "Is your foot bothering you?" It is also important to realize that some older persons may have language impairments that make it difficult to accurately identify the body part in pain. For example, in our bathing study we observed a woman who called out, "Ow! Don't touch my arm, it hurts," each time a nurse's aide moved her legs. The nurse's aide would argue that she was not touching her arm, because she really wasn't. Careful consultation with the nurse practitioner revealed that this woman had a history of stroke with resulting aphasia (language impairment). She also had severe diabetes with possible peripheral neuropathy (nerve pain) in her legs. Once this was known by the nurse's aide, she approached the woman more gently and informed her before moving her legs. This decreased the woman's need to call out about her "arms." In cases where language impairment is a problem, you may need to point to the body part you are assessing. Sometimes it takes patience and perseverance to find the best pain descriptor that makes sense to the person with dementia.

Assessment of Nonverbal Indicators of Pain

Assessment of nonverbal indicators of pain can be challenging, especially if you are not familiar with the person. However, there are reliable signals that have proven to be helpful in detecting discomfort (Table 6.3). The assessment of facial indicators of pain, like grimacing, can be more difficult in older persons because of wrinkles, oral tardive dyskinesia (repetitive mouth movements), and decreased clarity of facial expressions in end-stage dementia (Asplund, Norberg, Adolfsson, &

Waxman, 1991). Thus, facial expression alone should NOT be used to evaluate the presence of pain. It is also important to realize that there may not be vital sign changes associated with chronic pain, so that vital signs should NOT be used as an indicator of the presence or absence of pain.

Caregiver Wisdom

I know my patients very well and can usually tell if something is wrong. I look at their face for signs of pain such as a frown. Or they might be holding a part of their body. I sit and talk with them then and ask if they're hurting and try to get them to point to where it hurts. If they can't talk they might holler or scream. I get the nurse right away.

Edith Durham, CNA, Brian Center of Clayton, NC

Vocalizations of discomfort such as "Ow!, ouch!, or moaning" are important indicators that are often dismissed by hurried caregivers. Guarding, flinching, or rubbing a body part are other important behavioral indicators of pain that can provide data about need for pain treatment. Attention to these symptoms when they first present themselves can help the person be more comfortable and help you to protect yourself from injury during bathing.

TABLE 6.3   Nonverbal Indicators of Discomfort/Pain

frowning
eyes closing
nose wrinkling
squinting
fidgeting
tearfulness
noisy breathing
crying
grimacing
wincing
moaning
holding body stiffly
pushing caregiver away
hitting
yelling
pinching
high-pitched noises
resisting movements

Behavioral Symptoms

Many of the behavioral symptoms often seen during bathing such as hitting, pinching, and pushing the caregiver away may be attempts to stop movements that are producing pain. This is where your work as detective in determining whether there is a history of pain, current pain-causing conditions, and assessment of nonverbal pain indicators will provide clues as to whether pain is the underlying problem. It may be enough to change your approach to the person during bathing. However, sometimes the only way to be sure that pain is not causing behavioral symptoms is to do a trial of pain management and monitor the person's response. If behavioral symptoms decrease in response to adequate pain treatment then you can safely assume that it was an important cause of the behavioral symptoms for that person. It is also important to remember that the medications used for pain often have far fewer side effects than many psychiatric medications, like haloperidol, that are often given to people with dementia.

Cultural and Ethnic Issues in Pain Assessment

The expression and recognition of pain may vary by culture and ethnicity. Some cultural groups, such as Mexican-Americans, Ethiopians, and Japanese, place a strong value on stoicism or bearing pain without complaint (Lipson, Dibble, & Minarik, 1996). Many cultural groups, such as African-Americans, Eritreans, and Japanese-Americans, may have strong fears of addiction to pain medications and require extra support in taking medications (Lipson et al., 1996). Other cultures may encourage the sharing of body sensations, like pain. It is important to take culture and ethnicity into consideration during pain assessment, but individual differences are often more important than broad categorizations about ethnic differences. The most important thing is to individualize your assessment and treatment plan to the individual's unique values and needs.

Interventions to Minimize Pain During Bathing

Many things can be done to reduce the amount of pain experienced by persons with dementia during bathing. These include the way the person is approached and touched, environmental factors, nonmedication pain treatments, and the use of medications. Chapters 2, 4, and 10 describe many ideas for reducing pain. Additional methods for reducing pain are described below.

Nonmedication Treatments

There are several ways to reduce pain without using medications. Remember that some older people (and young ones too!) find a long hot soak in a tub is a good way to relieve pain, especially bone and muscle pain. How many of us have found a nice long soak in the tub helpful in reducing pain after activities like gardening or chopping firewood? Some urologists recommend a bath with 1/2 cup of baking soda added to reduce pain due to infections and conditions of the bladder. Encouraging an older adult to take a bath to relieve pain may help to reduce their reluctance to enter the bath. It is important to allow the person to relax in the bath and not rush him or her, especially if the bath is being used to minimize pain.

Many people get some relief from pain by using salves or ointments. You might offer to use some ointment to loosen up joints before a bath, or promise some extra ointment after a bath. This gives the person something to look forward to and helps him or her know that you want to make him or her more comfortable. However, some older adults with dementia have a hard time with irritant ointments, like capsaicin, because they have trouble interpreting why their skin is burning. Other people find that using a heat pack or a cold pack can reduce pain. You might need to experiment to find ways that help to relieve pain.

Complementary treatments like acupuncture and massage can help people with chronic pain conditions. These treatments have not been as well studied as medicines but they show real promise for treating pain. We saw a man who had very severe arthritis—so bad that his hands were all curled up. It was very difficult for his care providers to bathe and dress him, because he would become very upset, hit people, and try to stay in bed. A massage therapist began to treat him with gentle massage, initially for a few minutes at a time. Eventually, with the help of some medications too, his pain became much better managed, his hands opened up, and he stopped fighting his caregivers. The massage had a noticeable impact on his hitting people, and it seemed to his caregivers that he was much more comfortable after his massages.

Other cultures often add herbs like lavender or mint to a bath to reduce pain and discomfort. While there is limited research on this, it can make the bath more pleasurable. The nice thing about nonmedication pain treatment strategies is that they often have few side effects but real benefits for people with dementia.

Medication Management

Finding just the right dose and schedule of pain medication may be a process of experimentation to find the best relief with limited side effects. We recommend that clinicians rely on the American Geriatrics Society (AGS) Guidelines for the treatment of pain in older persons (American Geriatrics Society Panel on Chronic Pain in Older Persons, 1998). This paper provides guidelines on the state of the art for pain treatment according to experts in the care of older adults. The AGS suggests that medications be individually prescribed and increased depending on each person's response and side effects. As with other drugs for older adults, the adage "start low and go slow" (that is, starting a pain medication at a lower than normal dose and increasing it slowly) will reduce the risks associated with drug treatments.

The AGS guidelines recommend starting with a non-narcotic analgesic like acetaminophen, moving to narcotic analgesics if nonnarcotics are not effective, and increasing the dose or potency of narcotics until you get satisfactory pain relief. Most people find that the sedative (sleepiness) effects of narcotic pain medications wear off after a short time. Adjuvant drugs, or drugs used with analgesics, may help reduce pain. Some common adjuvant drugs used in treating chronic pain are antidepressant and anticonvulsant medications. Medications like aspirin or nonsteroidal anti-inflammatory drugs like ibuprofen often have too high a risk for older adults with multiple health problems and should not be used in general.

It is very important to start a constipation prevention (bowel) program when an older adult starts to take narcotic pain medication. Increasing fluid intake is an important part of any constipation prevention program. Many people get constipation from these drugs and use of a laxative can prevent unnecessary discomfort from these medications. For many older adults with limited mobility, bulking agents like Metamucil can cause uncomfortable bloating. Constipation is usually not a reason to stop pain medication. Work with the health care provider to find a bowel program that addresses the persons needs.

Timing the medication. Providing medications on a routine basis (around the clock) is the best way to provide consistent pain relief. The use of regularly scheduled medications prevents high and low levels of medication in the person's system and avoids breakthrough pain. Of course, the timing of the drugs should be guided by the person's schedule rather than the institution's. An example of a problem with this was when one resident was woken daily at 6:00 a.m. for pain medication because the day shift wanted the night nurse to give the medicine. The person often refused the medicine because they were too sleepy to understand what was happening. The night nurse, tired of arguing with the person, asked to have the medicine discontinued. Instead the medication time was changed to 8:00 a.m., the time when the person usually woke up, and there were no further problems with refusing the medicine.

If the person has only occasional pain with movement, it may be appropriate to provide pain medication 30–60 minutes before the bath. This helps to minimize the discomfort associated with all the activities required to get to the bath—undressing, transferring to the bath, getting washed and dried, and finally getting dressed again. It has been our experience, however, that this works better in home care settings than in institutional settings, where it can be difficult to organize medication administration with bathing times. Poorly timed medication can result in the person not getting sufficient pain relief to make bathing a more comfortable and pleasurable experience.

Medications to avoid in older adults. There are certain medications that are not recommended for use in older adults because of their risk of undesirable effects. Table 6.4 lists pain medications to avoid, since there are many safer, more effective alternatives (Beers, 1997). Often a geriatrician or geriatric nurse practitioner can help you chose the safest drugs for the person you are caring for. At times a pain specialist or pain clinic may be helpful if you are having a hard time treating the pain adequately and managing side effects. The most important thing to remember is that pain can be treated so the person's quality of life is better.

Collaboration With Others

Some health care providers may need to be convinced that an older person is having pain. You can do this by

TABLE 6.4 Pain and Related Medications to Avoid in Older Adults (Beers, 1997)

Trade Name	Generic Name	Reason to Avoid
Darvocet	Propoxyphene	No more effective than acetaminophen but with risks for falls, liver dysfunction
Demerol	Meperidine	Poor effects on pain, risk for delirium and falls
Indocin	Indomethacin	High risk for gastric problems and delirium
Butazolidin	Phenylbutazone	High risk for gastric problems, delirium, falls, and bone marrow depression
Talwin	Pentazocine	May precipitate pain crisis due to blockade of morphine-like receptors
Elavil	Amitriptyline	High risk for delirium, falls, constipation, urine retention, psychosis
Sinequan	Doxepin	High risk for delirium, falls, constipation, urine retention, psychosis
Librium	Chlordiazepoxide	High risk for delirium, falls, constipation, and physical dependence
Valium	Diazepam	High risk for delirium, falls, constipation, and physical dependence
Miltown	Meprobamate	High risk for delirium, falls, constipation, and physical dependence
All Barbiturates	Phenobarbital, Secobarbital, etc.	High risk for delirium, falls, constipation, and physical dependence

keeping track of pain reports, frequency of behaviors, and how they have responded to treatment with heat and simple over the counter medications like acetaminophen. You must present this information as data in a confident manner so that you can be an effective advocate for pain treatment. Some nurses have suggested that it is helpful to talk about a "pain crisis" when making calls to providers. This encourages the provider to call back promptly and to recognize that untreated pain really is a crisis to the person who suffers from it. Family members often have critical information about the person's pain history, usual style of coping with pain, and things that have and have not worked in the past to relieve pain. It is important for health care providers to work with family members as allies in making sure that pain is adequately treated in persons with dementia. Ask the family member the following questions:

- How does he/she usually express pain?
- Are there medications that have helped the pain in the past?
- Are there pain medications that he/she hasn't been helped by in the past?
- Does he/she use heat packs or ointments to help relieve pain?
- Are there any other things we should know about his/her pain?

If you are the family member of a person with dementia who you think is having pain, make a list before you call the doctor or nurse practitioner. Have the answers to the above questions ready so that you can give the provider enough information to make suggestions. You may want to try using acetaminophen for a few days before you call the provider to see if it makes a difference. You may need to advocate for the person with dementia. Don't take "no" for an answer if you believe pain is causing the battle with bathing.

REFERENCES

American Geriatrics Society, Panel on Chronic Pain in Older Persons. (1998). The management of chronic pain in older persons: AGS Panel on chronic pain in older persons. *Journal of the American Geriatrics Society, 46*(5), 635–651.

Asplund, K., Norberg, A., Adolfsson, R., & Waxman, H. (1991). Facial expressions in severely demented patients—a stimulus response study of four patients with dementia of the Alzheimer type. *International Journal of Geriatric Psychiatry, 6*, 599–606.

Bates, M., Rankin-Hill, L., & Sanchez-Ayendez, M. (1997). The effects of cultural context of health care on treatment of and response to chronic pain and illness. *Social Science & Medicine, 45*(9), 1433–1447.

Beers, M. (1997). Explicit criteria for determining potentially inappropriate medication use by the elderly: An update. *Archives of Internal Medicine, 157*(14), 1531–1536.

Feldt, K. S., Ryden, M. B., & Miles, S. (1998). Treatment of pain in cognitively impaired compared with cognitively intact older patients with hip fracture. *Journal of the American Geriatrics Society, 46*(9), 1079–1085.

Ferrell, B. A., Ferrell, B. R., & Osterweil, D. (1990). Pain in the nursing home. *Journal of the American Geriatrics Society, 38*(4), 409–414.

Ferrell, B. A., Ferrell, B. R., & Rivera, L. (1995). Pain in cognitively impaired nursing home patients. *Journal of Pain and Symptom Management, 10*(8), 591–598.

Galloway, S., & Turner, L. (1999). Pain assessment in older adults who are cognitively impaired. *Journal of Gerontological Nursing, 25*(7), 34–39.

Horgas, A. L., & Tsai, P. F. (1998). Analgesic drug prescription and use in cognitively impaired nursing home residents [see comments]. *Nursing Research, 47*(4), 235–242.

Kaasalainen, S., Middleton, J., Knezacek, S., Hartley, T., Stewart, N., Ife, C., & Robinson, L. (1998). Pain and cognitive status. *Journal of Gerontological Nursing, 24*(8), 24–31.

Kovach, C. R., Weissman, D. E., Griffie, J., Matson, S., & Muchka, S. (1999). Assessment and treatment of discomfort for people with late-stage dementia. *Journal of Pain & Symptom Management, 18*(6), 412–419.

Lipson, J., Dibble, S., & Minarik, P. (1996). *Culture and nursing care: A pocket guide.* San Francisco: UCSF Nursing Press.

Marzinski, L. R. (1991). The tragedy of dementia: Clinically assessing pain in the confused nonverbal elderly. *Journal of Gerontological Nursing, 17*(6), 25–28.

APPENDIX

Try the McGill Present Pain Intensity Questionnaire to assess the amount of pain a person is experiencing. This is the most widely used pain measure in clinical care. Photocopy the form and take it with you when you interview the person. Ask the person: "Are you uncomfortable now?" If the person is experiencing pain, show him or her the form and say: "Show me how uncomfortable you are now." You may have to try this several times before the person is able to use it appropriately.

Relevant Resources or Supplies

Clinical Practice Guidelines on the Management of Chronic Pain in Older Adults from the American Geriatric Society (AGS, 1998).

Adequate adaptive cushions for wheelchairs, lifts, and bathing chairs (see chapter 10)

Websites on pain:

Website of American Pain Society, an interdisciplinary organization.
http://www.ampainsoc.org/

Worldwide Congress on Pain; offers pain library and other services.
http://www.pain.com/

American Academy of Pain Management.
http://www.aapainmanage.org/

American Chronic Pain Association self-help group for chronic pain management.
http://members.tripod.com/~Widdy/ACPA.html

The Mayday Pain Project—has links to many other excellent pain websites.
http://www.painandhealth.org/

McGill Pain Questionnaire
Present Pain Inventory (PPI)

0 = No Pain

1 = Mild

2 = Discomforting

3 = Distressing

4 = Horrible

5 = Excruciating

Printed by permission of the author, Ronald Melzach, PhD.

CHAPTER 7

Care of the Skin

Johannah Topps Uriri, Kimberly Horton Hoffman,
and LouAnn Rondorf-Klym

As we age, we are more susceptible to skin problems because of normal aging changes in the skin and the immune system. For example, the skin may become dryer and more fragile, and thus more susceptible to tears and cracking. The first line of defense against infection is intact skin. However, breakdown of the skin can occur with prolonged exposure to water, use of excessive soap, and contact with urine and feces. The risk of infection increases once the skin breaks down, especially if the older person's immune system is compromised. Bathing procedures can be modified to help maintain the integrity of the skin and to decrease the risk of skin problems and infections. This chapter describes skin problems that may occur in older persons and body areas most vulnerable to these conditions. A procedure for checking the skin and infection control issues related to bathing are described. Finally, recommendations for preventive skin care are outlined.

Skin Characteristics

The normal skin of light-skinned older adults is dry, wrinkled, fragile, and sometimes yellowish. Other common effects of aging include wrinkling, sagging, blemishes, and freckle-like spots called age spots (lentigines). Exposed areas such as the elbows, knees, and the bottom of the feet may have rough areas. Some flaking or scaling is normal to see, but not excessive scaling and flaking or widespread roughness. Dark skin may be normally dry, flaky, and ashen in color.

The older adult's skin should be checked routinely for skin problems, such as scaling or flaking, cracking or skin tears, redness, rash, moist skin, and debris. Problematic skin areas may appear reddened (e.g., infections, pressure ulcers), hypopigmented (lighter) in white skin, or hyperpigmented (darker) in black skin. Gentle washing of the skin with soap and water is the primary means of removing body substances and other debris from the skin such as urine, feces and perspiration that can cause odor and irritate the skin. However, skin problems can occur or worsen because of the methods and procedures used during bathing. For example:

- Soap products left on the skin may result in dry and irritated skin.
- Improper drying may lead to skin tears and/or fungal infections.
- Areas left unwashed may result in skin irritations.
- Rash or infection may result from an allergic reaction to soap products.

The six most common skin problems associated with bathing and the possible causes of these problems are summarized in Table 7.1.

Skin Assessment

Persons with dementia can be more susceptible to skin problems if their hygiene is difficult to maintain. As a caregiver, you will need to pay special attention to the person's skin to ensure that skin problems do not develop, or are recognized and treated early. To prevent added distress, the best time to look at the skin is during the bath when the person is already undressed. Observe

TABLE 7.1   Skin Problems Associated With Bathing

Skin Problems	Definition	Possible Causes
Scaling or flaking	Small thin dandruff-like flakes of dried or dead skin	Soap
Cracking or skin tears	Skin resembles dried earth; slight cracking appearance may progress to tears in the skin.	Soap
Redness, hyperpigmentation or hypopigmentation	Pinkish to bright red or scarlet in color. In darker skin, the skins may appear much darker, purple or ashen gray when compared with surrounding skin.	Soap, allergies or infection
Rash	Bumps containing fluid may be intact, or weeping and crusting.	Infection, allergies, scabies
Moist skin (Maceration)	Skin looks thickened and white with boggy appearance. Boggy areas may have breaks in the skin (like a broken bubble).	Body parts not completely dried or sweating
Foreign body debris	Dirt, liquid, or food spills, body substances (dried blood, spit, stool, urine), or dead skin cells between toes.	Poor hygiene

the chest, upper arms, stomach area, underneath the arms, back, inner thighs, groin creases, genital and rectal areas, upper and lower legs, feet, and between the toes for skin problems. Check for skin problems described in Table 7.1. Look carefully as you assist the person with washing and drying each part of the body. Become familiar with the person's skin so that you can observe changes before they become serious problems. How often this should occur will vary with the person's health and skin condition.

The best procedure is to:

- Wash your hands with soap and warm water and dry your hands.
- Provide for privacy and keep the person warm at all times.
- Look carefully at the skin when you are removing the person's clothing.
- Check each body area as you wash the skin.
- Rinse the soap away completely (unless using a no-rinse solution).
- Before drying, check skin folds for soap (underneath the arms, breasts, and abdomen; in the groin creases, genital and rectal areas; between the toes).
- Continue to look closely at the skin as you pat the skin dry.
- Check to ensure that the skin folds are dry.
- Check carefully as you dry between the toes.

- Tell the health care provider, charge nurse, or other appropriate person about any changes you notice.

Caregiver Wisdom

With our residents you have to wash the skin very gently. Make sure you put lotion on it every day 'cause their skin is so dry. I check for red marks when I do a.m. care and as I dry them after a bath.

Edith Durham, CNA, Brian Center of Clayton, NC

Observing in a comprehensive manner the skin of individuals who are very private, dislike having parts of the body touched, or are getting a towel bath in which the skin is not as exposed, may be difficult. In these situations, try examining the skin while assisting the person during toileting. You will need to use your ingenuity and skill to assure that adequate observation occurs and potential problems are discovered and addressed early.

Infection Control

Infection control is the sum total of the effort to keep the person's environment free of potential pathogenic microorganisms such as bacteria and fungi that the normal defenses of an older person's body may be less able to fight. Environmental factors such as cross-contamination associated with equipment used during tub baths and showers in shared bathing facilities can contribute to infections. Medications (e.g., antibiotics, immunosuppressants) that change the skin flora contribute to the natural selection of pathogenic organisms. Transient organisms and overgrowth of microflora can become a problem for older adults under these conditions. Thus, basic infection control knowledge is important to prevent infections from occurring and to control infections that are already present.

As a caregiver, you can help prevent the transfer of infection to yourself or others by following these guidelines during bathing activities:

- Keep dirty and clean items separate.
- If a clean item becomes dirty, get a new clean item.
- Bathe the person from the 'cleanest' areas to the 'dirtiest' areas when possible or use different washcloths for different body parts to reduce the spread of microorganisms to cleaner areas of the body.
- Clean bathing areas after each use with a cleaning agent containing chlorine.
- If the person has an obvious infection, open wound, or pressure ulcer, wear gloves and a waterproof gown when bathing or providing care.

As a caregiver, you can help prevent the growth of microorganisms on the skin following these guidelines during bathing activities:

- Use tepid water.
- Use a small amount of soap.
- Wash skin gently.
- Rinse soap completely (unless using no-rinse soap).
- Keep skin folds (underneath breast, groin, axilla) dry.
- Keep skin lubricated.

Assess medications and use extra care when the person is taking medications that change the skin flora (e.g., antibiotics or immunosuppressive drugs).

To prevent and control infections when using a bed bath or basin bath procedure, precautions such as washing hands, using gloves, and protecting clothes with a gown are important also. Generally, wash from the least soiled area to the most soiled area (head, face, neck, upper arms, abdomen, upper and lower legs, and feet). Then, change the washcloth and water (if using a basin) and wash the most soiled areas (genitalia to rectum). If this general approach is distressing to the person it can be safely and skillfully modified to meet personal needs and preferences.

Approaches to Skin Care to Prevent Skin Problems

To prevent excessive dryness that may be caused by soap products, the chest, upper arms, upper and lower legs, and abdomen should be washed with a small amount of lotion and water (a couple of squirts of lotion into a basin of warm water). These areas usually are not contaminated with urine, feces, or perspiration. Mild soap such as Dove that contains fats or a gentle no-rinse soap substitute solution can be used underneath the arms and in the groin, genital, and rectal areas. These areas are more likely to become contaminated with urine or feces, or to trap moisture and organisms that can contribute to odor. Rinse off the soap completely unless you are using a no-rinse solution. Always check the areas for allergic reactions (e.g., redness, swelling, rash) to the cleansing product. Pat the skin dry instead of rubbing and apply lubricants after drying the skin.

Caregiver Wisdom

I've been a nursing assistant for 7 years. I've learned that if a person doesn't like a shower, you need to try a Keri™ or sponge bath. They smell great and their skin is much better. It's easier to get them clean and you don't need a lot of water.
Terri Johnson, CNA, Hillcrest Convalescent Center, Durham, NC

To prevent moisture-related problems, check to be sure that the skin folds are dry. To prevent acne in black skin, products such as lanolin, petroleum jelly (Vaseline™), vegetable oils, or waxes should be avoided. Instead, use small amounts of olive or fish

TABLE 7.2 Preventing and Addressing Skin Problems

Skin Problems	Prevention/Action
Scaling or flaking	Superfatted soap and tepid water. Control humidity in the environment. Lubricants and moisturizers or hydrogenated vegetable (e.g., Eucerin™, Keri Lotion™ or oil, hydrogenated Crisco™).
Ash	Moisturizers (e.g., small amount of olive oil or fish oil, Keri Lotion™ or oil).
Cracking or skin tears	Lubricants and moisturizers. Hemorrhoid preparation (e.g., Preparation H™ is good for rough areas on the soles of the foot, elbows, and ankles).
Redness	Rinse area completely, and contact the person's health care provider for treatment of allergies and scabies.
Rash	Contact the person's health care provider for the treatment of allergies and scabies.
Moisture	Make sure skin folds are cleansed and dried completely and apply cornstarch to keep the areas dry.
Foreign body debris	Clean body areas adequately.

oils or moisturizing oils such as Keri oil to moisturize black skin. Hemorrhoid preparations (Preparation H™ or a generic brand) that include shark liver oil as an ingredient can be used for wrinkles and rough spots or cracking on the soles of the feet, elbows, knees, and ankles. Table 7.2 describes interventions that can be used to prevent or address skin problems.

Conclusion

The skin of older adults is fragile and requires special attention and care during bathing to prevent skin breakdown and bacterial or fungal infections. Individuals diagnosed with dementia are at greater risk for these problems; therefore it is important for caregivers to provide extra care when assisting during bathing. Check the person's skin routinely, during undressing, bathing, and toileting activities. Report any changes to a health care provider who can assist you in correcting skin problems. Preventing infection is important during bathing to avoid further problems that may cause harm to the person being bathed, to yourself, and to others with whom you may come in contact after the bath. Also, pay special attention to soap products because it is important to select products that are not irritating to the skin. Make sure the skin is clean and dry, especially the folds of the skin. The use of moisturizing products can be helpful in reducing skin problems that are associated with bathing. Following the procedures described in this chapter can prevent skin problems that are seen

frequently in clinics, hospitals, nursing homes, and in the home setting.

REFERENCES

Brown, D., & Sears, M. (1993). Perineal dermatitis: A conceptual framework. *Ostomy and Wound Management, 39*(7), 20–22.

Fordyce, M. (1999). *Geriatric PEARLS* (pp. 6, 14). Philadelphia: F. A. Davis Company.

Hardy, M. A. (1990). A pilot study of the diagnosis and treatment of impaired skin integrity: Dry skin in older persons. *Nursing Diagnosis, 1*(2), 57–63.

Hardy, M. A. (2001). Impaired skin integrity: Dry skin. In M. L. Mass, T. Tripp-Reimer, K. C. Buckwalter, M. Titler, M. D. Hardy, & J. P. Specht (Eds.), *Nursing care of older adults* (pp. 137–144). St. Louis: Mosby, Inc.

Johnson, B. L., Moy, R. L., & White, G. M. (1998). *Ethnic skin, medical and surgical* (pp. 32–40). St. Louis: Mosby, Inc.

Kovach, T. (1988). Controlling infection as part of the bath process. *Provider, 14*(12), 43–44.

Leyden, J. J., McGingley, K. J., Norstrom, K. M., & Webster, G. F. (1987). Skin microflora. *The Journal of Investigative Dermatology, 88*(3), 65s–72s.

Lueckenotte, A. G. (1994). *Pocket guide to gerontologic assessment* (pp. 60–81). St. Louis: Mosby.

Montagna, W., Prota, G. P., & Kennedy, J. A. (1993). *Black skin structure and function* (pp. 132–133). San Diego: Academic Press.

Patterson, J. A. K. (1989). *Aging and clinical practice: Skin disorders.* New York: Igaku-Shoin.

Roth, R. R., & James, W. D. (1989). Microbiology of the skin: Resident flora, ecology, infection. *Journal of the American Academy of Dermatology, 20*(3), 367–481.

Wysocki, A. B., & Bryant, R. A. (1992). Skin. In R. Bryant (Ed.), *Acute and chronic wounds nursing management* (pp. 1–30). St. Louis: Mosby-Year Book, Inc.

CHAPTER 8

Transfer Techniques

Adele Mattinat Spegman, Theresa H. Raudsepp,
and Jennifer R. Wood

Many frail elders require assistance getting from their beds to the sink, tub or shower. For some, it necessitates getting out of bed and walking. But for many, bath time encompasses multiple transfers: in and out of bed, to the wheelchair or shower chair, on and off the toilet or commode. Such physical activity provides many benefits to the bather but also introduces risks of injury to both the elderly person and the caregiver. This chapter describes methods of safely and effectively assisting these transfers. Transfers are regarded as therapeutic when respecting the comfort, need, and dignity of the person, while protecting caregivers from injury. Such an approach has direct applicability not only to the bathing process, but also to caregiving in general.

This chapter is divided into five sections. First, the importance of this topic is reviewed, both for the person being assisted and for ourselves as caregivers. The next section reviews the essential foundations of successful transfers: good body mechanics, safety considerations, and cueing the person being transferred. Then we present strategies for assessing and choosing a transfer method. The fourth section describes specific transfer methods using diagrams and illustrations. The chapter ends with a discussion of how to make therapeutic transfers a routine practice.

Why Safe Transfer Techniques Are Important

The transfer technique should be regarded as a prescription for the best means of mobility for the person, keeping in mind the person's functional capabilities. If at all possible, transfers should involve some weight-bearing movements. Such movements facilitate muscle strength and range of motion in joints, improve circulation, maintain bone density, and increase alertness. Osteoporosis is slowed by weight-bearing through the long bones of the arms and legs. Furthermore, active participation in one's care and comfort is linked to increased self-esteem.

The "underarm" method of helping is popular but dangerous for both the person being cared-for and the caregiver (Figures 8.1 and 8.2). First, it can cause caregiver injury by straining the lower back (Garg & Owen, 1992). For the person being assisted, the underarm method is a painful way of preventing a fall and potentially causes other injuries, such as bruising, muscle strains, nerve trauma, and shoulder dislocation (Owen & Carlson, 1992). In 1992 the underarm method was reported to be used in 98% of manual lifting transfers (Garg & Owen, 1992), and in a 1994 survey was witnessed by 94% of nurses and taught by 83% of the nursing instructors (Owen, Welden, & Kane, 1999). We must modify our transfer practices if we strive to provide quality care!

Mechanical lifts are being used to minimize the risk of caregiver injuries. In fact, some long-term care facilities have a "zero-lift" policy so staff do not directly lift any residents. Yet the mechanical lifts do not eliminate staff injuries. Conversely, use of these devices does reduce the opportunities for and benefits of active weight-bearing transfers. Furthermore, using lifts to transfer people with dementia may heighten their confusion, anxiety, and resistance to the transfer.

Unfortunately, caregivers often direct their attention to the mechanical device instead of the person being transferred. Wood and Raudsepp, for example, found that caregivers communicated less during transfers when mechanical lifts were used in comparison with

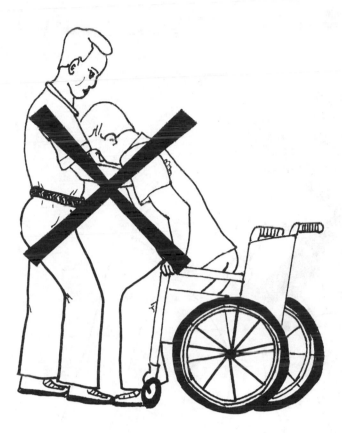

FIGURE 8.1 Incorrect underarm transfer method—1 caregiver.

transfer approaches without such devices. Thus, although lifts are a valuable tool for safe transfers, the use of mechanical devices is not a panacea and requires careful consideration of the pros and cons in each individual case.

Caregiver Wisdom

Some places I have worked have a no-lift policy. There is a better way. Our techniques are safe for the staff and allow people to use as much of their abilities as possible.
Janine Nelson, CNA, CMA, Providence
Benedictine Nursing Center, Mt. Angel, OR

The Basics of Safe Transfers

Three issues are fundamental to all successful transfer techniques:

- good body mechanics
- attention to safety
- cueing the person being transferred.

Optimal body mechanics includes the positioning of both caregiver and person being transferred. Safe techniques require that we be aware of how to efficiently use available resources: equipment, other caregivers, and a variety of transfer techniques. Most important, consistent technique and clear communication maximize the person's participation and decrease anxiety.

The Basics of Body Mechanics

Take care of yourself! The job description of a caregiver requires flexibility, strength, and stamina. It has been described as one of the most dangerous professions in America due to the high incidence of back injuries. Good body mechanics is a first defense towards preventing injury (Table 8.1). As caregivers, we are responsible for achieving a fitness level that meets the physical demands of caregiving activities. Some of the caregiving physical demands include:

- tolerance of repeated bending and stooping.
- ability to lift 50 lbs. while maintaining good body mechanics.

TABLE 8.1 Examples of Good Body Mechanics

1. Bend knees and lift with legs.
2. Keep back vertical, maintaining the three natural curves.
3. Avoid overreaching with arms, keep shoulder blades pulled back.
4. Tighten abdominal muscles during lift.
5. Avoid twisting the back.
6. Pivot feet with body when turning.
7. Get close to the load.
8. Lower your center of gravity for the lift.
9. Communicate with your lifting partner, and the person being lifted.
10. Get a second person if you feel uncomfortable.
11. Plan ahead and secure all the equipment.
12. Test the load before lifting.
13. Do not complete the lift if it doesn't feel safe.
14. Counterbalance the load by shifting your weight back to decrease strain.
15. When working over the bed, put the rail down and knee on the bed.

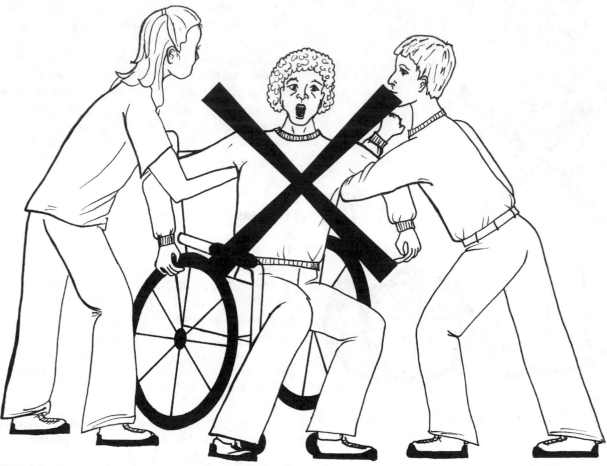

FIGURE 8.2   Incorrect underarm transfer method—2 caregivers.

- ability to fully squat.
- ability to kneel on one or both knees.

Bedside Body Mechanics

Caregiving activities often involve frail and disabled people in bed. Our backs are vulnerable to injury with prolonged leaning and bending when providing bedside care. The good news is that the use of body mechanics can be tailored to bedside care! The following tips limit back strain when caregiving for people in bed:

- Put down or remove the bed rails on the side you are working on.
- Place one knee on the bed when assisting a person in rolling or scooting in bed.
- Use a drawsheet under the person for leverage and comfort while moving in bed.

- If possible, adjust the bed height so that you are comfortable and avoid leaning over.
- When rolling a person over, have the person assist by first bending their knees up, then pulling on the siderail in the direction of the roll.
- When washing a person's back, position the person in bed lying face down, propped on pillows partway under the shoulder and hip. This position relieves the caregiver from having to physically hold the person with one hand while attempting to wash with the other.

Basic Safety Considerations

- *Plan ahead.* Think through the details of the transfer. Know what method to use and how many people are needed. Have all equipment needed

Special Concerns

close by. Know the person's physical and cognitive limitations, and which side to go to.

- *Equipment such as beds, wheelchairs, and shower chairs, needs to be in good working order.* This implies effective brakes, removable armrests, and adjustable height. Whenever possible, adjust the bed height so the transfer surfaces are equal, or make the second surface slightly lower to avoid transferring "uphill."

- *Stabilize equipment before a transfer.* Don't trust the "wheel brakes" on beds and shower chairs. Place them up against the wall or something heavy to keep them from moving during the transfer.

- *Recognize situations requiring the assistance of a second person.* If the person has poor trunk control and is unable to sit independently at the edge of the bed, a second caregiver will be needed to get behind and help with balance during the transfer. It is necessary for the second person assisting to get up onto the bed close to the person being lifted for good body mechanics. This second caregiver should assist under the person's buttocks, using a barrier such as a towel or chux to protect both the person and the caregiver. Gloves may be necessary when doing a shower transfer.

- *Use a transfer belt.* A regular belt with a buckle can also work. Place the belt low on the person's hips at a 45 degree angle from seat bottom. This position is more comfortable for the person and provides a more effective line of pull.

- *Always block the person's knee with your knee(s) from the moment he/she is at the edge of the bed, until he/she is all the way back on the chair.* This prevents the person from sliding forward off the surface, and helps prevent buckling during the transfer. The knee block should be IN FRONT of the person's knee and not squeezing it from both sides. It is recommended to only block one of the person's knees to control the transfer. If needed for comfort, a hand towel can be folded and placed against the knee for padding.

- *Never assist any person's transfer by pulling or holding on to his/her arms.* Serious injury to the shoulder joint of the person being lifted can occur, it is uncomfortable, and it gets in the way of the person's normal movement pattern.

- *Do not allow the person being transferred to hold on to the caregiver's neck, shoulders, or arms.* This can cause serious injury to the caregiver's neck and shoulders. If the person is unable to push up from the surface with his/her arms, as a last resort ask him/her to hold on to the caregiver's waistband, or belt. This often feels very secure to the person being transferred and is a safer option for the caregiver than holding onto the caregiver's neck or shoulders.

- *Do not undress the person during the transfer.* Do it before or after. The transfer is challenging enough without trying to manage clothing at the same time.

- *Be prepared for the unexpected.* There should always be a safe "way out" during the transfer should the person become unresponsive, combative, or frightened. The Scoot Method of transfer (described in the following section) allows the person to sit down even in the middle of a transfer, providing the caregiver with a chance to reposition for better body mechanics.

Communication Basics: Share Your Plans

A transfer can be a very traumatic experience for a person who is dependent. Multiple factors can come into play, heightening fear, anxiety, and pain. Cognitive impairment as well as poor eyesight and hearing, poor balance, vertigo, pain, and personal issues can affect the person's perception of a transfer. Anxiety can be compounded by the fact that during a bath transfer, the person is often unclothed, which may contribute to a heightened sense of vulnerability.

Thoughtful use of words and cues can improve the transfer experience for the person. Build trust by reassuring often, validating the person's feelings and concerns, and giving clear cues. Use the following strategies:

- *ALWAYS speak to the person at eye level.* This may mean squatting down. Eye contact is important.

- *Be flexible.* Give the person some choice as to time or method.

- *Adjust for deficits.* Ask the person if they would like to wear glasses and hearing aids during transfers. Gestures work very well for persons who are hard of hearing or cognitively impaired. A dry erase board can be used with persons who are deaf or cannot speak.

- *Explain who you are and the goal of the transfer.*
- *Appear as if you have all the time in the world.* Give the person ample time to react to your request—and do not start moving the person until you see them initiating the movement.
- *Invite the person to help you.* Most people will do all they can to help. Say "I would like to help you . . . " instead of "I am going to. . . . " This implies that the person is actively involved in the activity rather than having some procedure "done to him/her." Use words that connote security such as "hold on here" or "grab this for balance." Avoid words like "lean forward" and "move to the edge" that provoke anxiety in an anxious person. Instead, instruct the person to "put your head on my shoulder." Praise the person's efforts to help, no matter how small.
- *Smile often.*
- *Reassure the person that you will not let him/her fall.* Acknowledge that it is scary for him/her to move this way. Be sensitive about what is said in front of the person. For example, to avoid feelings of anxiety don't say "I've never done this before" or "My back is killing me today."
- *Keep directions short and simple.* If more than one caregiver is needed, designate which caregiver will be directing the person to avoid confusion and distraction.
- *Stop the transfer if the person becomes combative or terrified despite your reassurances.*

Choosing an Appropriate Transfer Method

The Transfer Progression Continuum (Figure 8.3) provides a visual reference for different types of transfer. They range from independent to dependent. As a person's needs change for better or worse, the appropriateness of the transfer method changes. The goal is to maintain the highest level of functioning and safety.

The choice of transfer varies according to the amount of aid required by the person and the number of caregivers assisting with the transfer. The best transfer method for a given situation reflects the person's physical abilities as well as behavioral, environmental, and resource issues (Table 8.2). There needs to be a balance between

TABLE 8.2 Choosing an Appropriate Transfer Method

The following questions are useful guides for choosing an appropriate transfer method.

1. What is the person's sitting balance? How much assistance does this person need to sit upright? Two caregivers may be needed to safely transfer a person with poor sitting balance.
2. What is the length of time that a person can comfortably sit? This assessment is important for pacing plans. A shorter sitting tolerance requires that the transfer be done with efficiency and advanced preparation.
3. What is the person's ability to stand and bear weight through the legs? Appropriate transfers for persons with poor weight-bearing abilities include the scoot, sliding board, or draw-sheet methods.
4. What is the person's skin tolerance to sitting on different surfaces? Assessing the skin's sensitivity is a first step in minimizing skin abrasions and tears. The next step is to adequately pad the surfaces of any equipment used in the transfer.
5. What type of equipment is necessary for the transfer and bathing technique? For example, will the person need a backrest or removable armrests or a bath blanket to pad the equipment (i.e., slideboard)?

---

assisting enough while not overassisting. Standard definitions have been developed:

- minimal assistance = person can assist 75%, caregiver must assist 25%
- moderate assistance = person can assist 50%, caregiver must assist 50%
- maximum assistance = person can assist 25%, caregiver must assist 75%

Assessing how much help the person needs allows caregivers to maintain the person's functional abilities and prevent injuries to the person and their caregiver.

The transfers identified down the continuum provide increasing caregiver assistance as dependence increases. The lateral movement (left > right) gives alternative choices dependent on specific situations and the number of available caregivers. For example, as a person with dementia experiences a decline, the transfer method will slide down the continuum when one caregiver assists with the transfer. Alternatively, the caregiver may choose a two-person assist in recognition of physical difficulties, behavioral issues, or an awkward environment.

An initial physical or occupational therapy consult should be obtained to determine the person's strength,

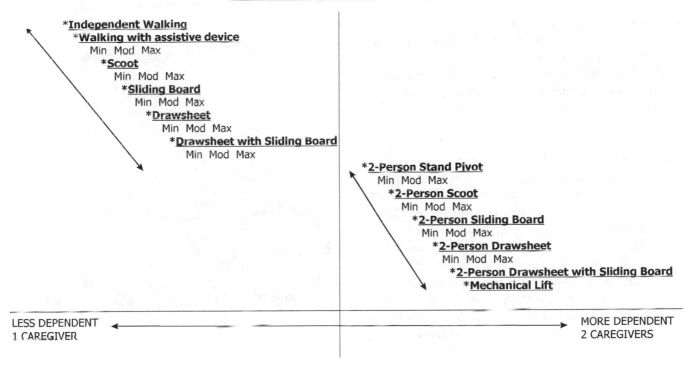

FIGURE 8.3 Transfer progression continuum.

Note: From *Transfer Training Program*, by T. H. Raudsepp & J. R. Wood, 1996, Mt. Angel, OR: Providence Benedictine Nursing Center. Copyright 1996 Theresa H. Raudsepp, Jennifer R. Wood, and Providence Benedictine Nursing Center. Reprinted with permission of the authors.

range of motion, and the safest transfer method. However, recognizing that changes in people's strength and health occur, you should examine the person's transfer needs on an ongoing basis.

Preparing the Person for the Transfer

The initial step in any transfer is preparation of the person. Follow these steps to get the elder to the "ready" position prior to every transfer:

- Have the person scoot forward to the edge of the seat to the point that they cannot see the chair or bed between their legs. This movement occurs by shifting weight onto one hip at a time. You can squat in front and assist from behind the person's hips as needed.

- Place the person's feet back so that their toes are directly under their knees.
- Ask the person to sit up straight and bend forward so that their shoulders are over their toes.
- Cue the person to push up from the surface with both hands, if able.

Develop a consistent cue so that the person knows when they are to move. It is helpful to use three rocking motions and the verbal cues "one, two, three," with movement occurring on "three." This rocking phase can help to relax people who are stiff and rigid and make leaning forward easier. You need to stay out of the person's normal movement pattern as much as possible.

Preparation eliminates unnecessary lifting. Cognitively impaired persons can better understand what it is they are supposed to be doing if you assist them into the "ready" position. This strategy also provides a weight-bearing opportunity.

Specific Transfer Methods

Walker transfer (Figure 8.4)

Purpose: This technique assists the person to stand, turn with the walker, then sit.

Skills: Use it with a person who has fair balance and is able to bear considerable weight through his/her arms and legs. Usually, one caregiver is required.

Procedure:

a.   Place a transfer belt around the person's waist. For optimal body mechanics, assist the person from the side and slightly behind, not the front. When a person with a walker loses their balance, they almost always fall backwards.

b.   Using verbal and physical cues, have the person push up to stand from the surface he/she is sitting on. Do not pull up on the walker since it can tip over. Once standing, have the person place his/her hands on the walker for balance. The person should then step around to the next sitting surface, backing up to this surface until both legs are touching the seat.

c.   Direct the person to bend forward and then reach backwards with both hands to touch the seat (or armrests). Now ask the person to sit down slowly bending knees in a controlled manner.

Stand pivot transfer (Figure 8.5)

Purpose: This technique assists the person to stand, turn without the walker, then sit.

Skills: Use only with a person who can bear weight while taking a few small steps.

Procedure:

a.   Place the transfer belt low on the person's hips. Stand in front of the person. Block the person's knees in the front by placing both of your knees against the person's.

b.   Holding on to the transfer belt and the person's hips, rock the person forward over his/her feet three times, counting "one, two, three." It is great to have the person being transferred do the counting aloud, as this allows him/her to direct the transfer, and assures he/she will be ready. Each rock should bring the person farther forward and up out of the seat. Sink very low, sitting back as if there is a chair behind you. Stay out of the person's way as they lean over their feet.

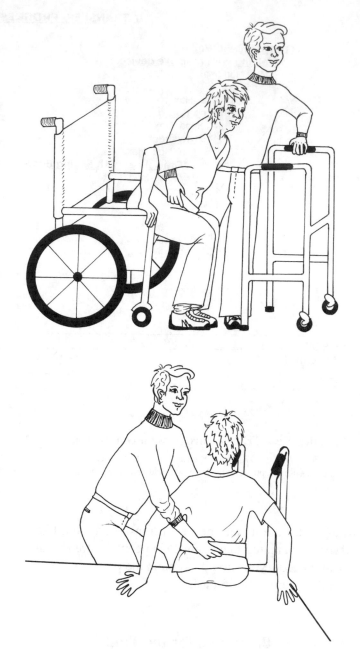

FIGURE 8.4   Walker transfer.

c.   On the third rock, assist the person to a full stand, supporting at the hips with the belt, and at the knee with the knee block. If necessary, the elder can hold the transfer belt around your waist.

d.   As the person gets balanced, both take small steps around, backing up to the second surface until both of the person's legs are touching the sitting surface.

e. Ask the person to lean forward and then reach back for the seat (or arms of the chair) with both arms, and sit down in a slow, controlled manner. Remain in close contact, blocking the person's knees throughout the transfer to prevent buckling.

Scoot transfer (Figure 8.6)

Purpose: assists the person to move from one sitting area to another in 2–3 small scoots as opposed to one pivot movement. This method protects your back from twisting during a lift. It is appropriate for transfers to bed, chair, commode, or shower chair. Remove armrests because small movements will occur and the person will not be lifted high enough to clear the armrest.

Skills: The Scoot Transfer requires little ability to help and prevents injury to the person's hips, knees, and ankles, which are vulnerable to twisting during the traditional stand pivot transfer. Anxiety in the person being transferred is decreased because the movements are smaller and slower. This method can be used as a one- or two-caregiver transfer.

Procedure: one caregiver

a. Place the transfer belt low on person's hips. Use a solid knee block throughout this transfer. Before the first scoot, determine the distance to be moved. Tell the person how many scoots are anticipated.

b. After rocking forward three times over their feet, the person is lifted slightly off the seating surface and is moved laterally just a few inches toward the second surface. A blanket or pad can be placed in the space between the two surfaces to protect the skin from the equipment. The person should be lifted only enough to clear the surface and to allow the hips to scoot sideways.

c. Continue the process two or more times until the person is seated all the way back on the second surface.

Procedure: two caregivers.

A second caregiver assists from behind when the person has poor trunk control. Cues are given by the first (front) caregiver to avoid confusion.

a. The second caregiver gets all the way up on the bed behind the person, using a barrier as needed. The second caregiver controls the person's trunk by keeping the shoulder midline and over the feet.

b. During the rocking phase, the second caregiver places his/her hands far under the person's hips to guide his/her hips. The transfer belt is not used by the second caregiver. He/she continues to control the person's trunk midline over the person's feet with his/her shoulders.

c. The two caregivers take turns repositioning themselves and the person after each scoot to maintain good body mechanics with the front caregiver maintaining the knee block on the person at all times.

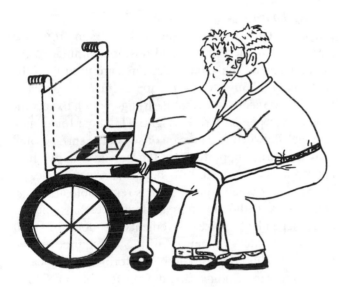

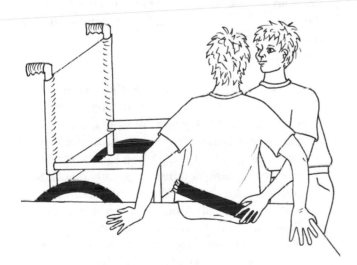

FIGURE 8.5 Stand pivot transfer.

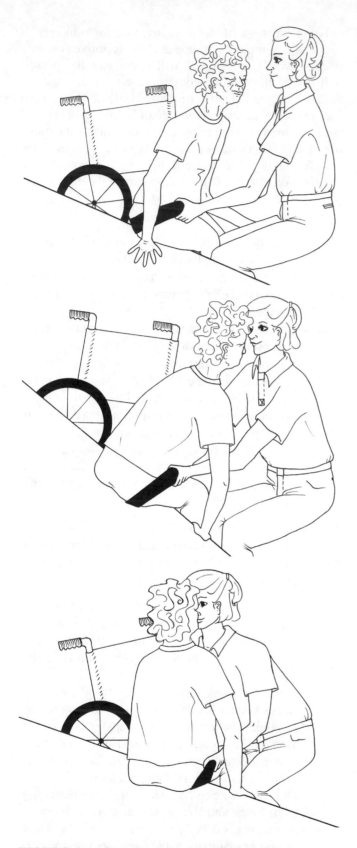

FIGURE 8.6   Scoot transfer, 1-caregiver assist.

Sliding board transfer (Figure 8.7)

Purpose: This technique slides the person from one surface to another, in a seated position. Similar to the Scoot Transfer, the same procedures are used with the addition of a laminated board approximately 10 inches wide by 20 inches long that is strong enough to accommodate the person's full weight. This board acts as a "bridge" between two uneven or separated surfaces and provides firm support under the person's body. It is appropriate for transfers to bed, chair, commode, or shower chair when equipment has removable armrests.

Skills: This method is often used with persons who are more dependent. Since movements are done in small scoots, a limited amount of lifting is required of the caregiver. This transfer can be performed with one or two caregivers. Sliding Board Transfers become difficult when the person is unclothed and wet and additional precautions are needed when the technique is used with baths. See Table 8.3 for suggestions for protecting the skin during transfers.

Procedure: one caregiver.

a. Place the transfer belt low on the person's hips.
b. Ask the person to lean to the opposite side. Carefully lift the leg upward from the knee, and place the board at an angle toward the "sit bones" or ischial tuberosities. Look and ask while doing this to be sure nothing is getting pinched or poked by the board. The sliding board should form a diagonal "bridge" under the person's thigh between the two transfer surfaces.
c. Rock the person three times, then guide the person as he/she scoots across the board.
d. Once the transfer is complete, remove the board. Have the person lean away; lift the leg and gently remove the board.

TABLE 8.3 Suggestions for Protecting Skin During Transfers

- Place a pillowcase or chux over sliding board before placing it.
- Use talc powder to make the surface slick and absorb skin moisture and reduce friction.
- An athletic supporter or "jockstrap" protects a man's genitals from being pinched while allowing the rectal area to be cleaned.
- A pillowcase can also be used to help hold the genitals up safely during the transfer, (placed between person's legs like a brief) and can be carefully removed and replaced through the hole in the shower chair.

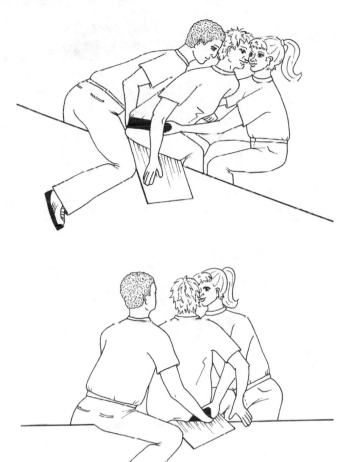

Procedure: two caregivers.

a. If a second caregiver is needed, he/she should assist from behind as described with the Scoot Method.

b. To keep the sliding board from moving during the transfer (usually the initial scoot), have the person or second caregiver stabilize the board with one hand flat on the board.

Looped drawsheet transfer (Figure 8.8)

Purpose: This is the ideal method when wearing a transfer belt may be uncomfortable for the person or contraindicated by medical issues, such as abdominal incision, feeding tube, or colostomy bag. A drawsheet replaces the transfer belt, providing a greater area of support to the person's hips and increasing comfort by dispersing pressure. The method works very well for transfers to commodes and shower chairs in which the person is not clothed. Armrests must be removed.

Skills: Use with persons who are more dependent. It can be done by one or two caregivers.

Procedure: one caregiver.

a. Bunch up a flat sheet, lengthwise, to form a long band 5-6 inches wide. Place this around the back of the pelvis of the seated person. Loop the sheet under the person's thighs in front, forming a "donut" for the person to sit on.

b. Pull the sheet around the person so it is very snug. One hand holds the sheet together at one side, even with the person's hip bones; the other hand holds the sheet looped in the same area on the other side. Leverage is provided via the snug sheet.

c. The transfer is performed in two or more small scoots, as described with the Scoot and Sliding Board Methods.

FIGURE 8.7   Sliding board transfer, 2-caregiver assist.

d. The sheet is removed easily as soon as the transfer is complete.

Procedure: two caregivers.

a. The second caregiver assists in the Looped Drawsheet Transfer just as in the Scoot and Sliding Board Transfers, working from behind the person, with hands under the person's hips. The second caregiver does not hold on to the sheet as this can make it slip.

Making Therapeutic Transfers Routine Practice

A comprehensive transfer training program is the most effective strategy for providing therapeutic transfers and

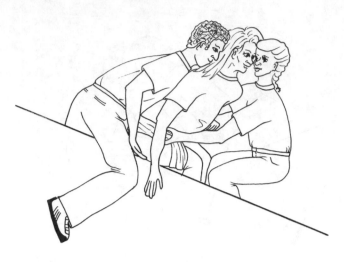

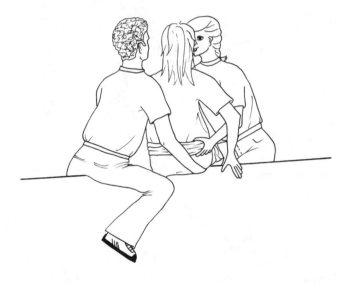

FIGURE 8.8 Looped drawsheet transfer, 2-caregiver assist.

minimizing the number and cost of caregiver injuries. This requires establishing policies, monitoring practices, and maintaining quality care and caregiver well-being. Suggestions for a transfer training protocol include:

- Make transfer classes MANDATORY for all who are connected with providing, supervising, or monitoring caregiving: CNAs, LPNs, RNs, medication technicians, supervisors, and resident care managers. Values, understandings, and expectations are more likely to be shared with an inclusive approach.

- Classes should be long enough to provide instruction and hands-on practice of transfer techniques by caregivers under the instructor's supervision.
- Provide both basic and advanced classes. Advanced classes should include role-playing of case examples and group problem-solving on difficult situations that arise with "real people." In this way, advanced classes become "case reviews" and "continuing education."
- Offer classes monthly, either as basic or advanced classes. Provide a consistent class synopsis to participants and require that those standards be followed on the floor.
- Momentum can be sustained using a variety of interventions, as described in Table 8.4.

TABLE 8.4 Strategies for Maintaining a System-Wide Transfer Program

Choose broad topics for inservice education programs	• "PROMOTE FITNESS!" Inservice staff on back exercises for improved posture and strength.
	• "The pros/cons of mechanical lifts and when and how to use them." Establish and discuss guidelines for carefully assessing need.
	• "Communicating with cognitively impaired people." Invite a geriatric or mental health specialist.
Attend to the needs of the caregiver	• Provide transfer belts for every person and *require* their use.
	• Survey the staff for feedback on effectiveness of transfer education.
Promote activities that involve unit-based teamwork	• Schedule floor inservices for residents presenting transfer challenges, encouraging RNs to problem-solve and assist CNAs at bedside transfer sessions.
	• Provide detailed instruction on individual transfer method for staff via wall signs and bedside information sheets.
	• Videotape difficult transfers being done properly and leave on unit for staff to review together.
Evaluate transfer method choices as a quality assurance program	• Use the transfer progression continuum to track the appropriateness of transfer methods for individual residents
	• Track incidents involving moving residents and caregiver work-related injuries and intervene where needed.
	• Communicate tracking results to all involved

Caregiver Wisdom

What I see happening in other places feels unsafe to me. It seems like throwing people into chairs with no warning. After learning these new techniques, I feel more in control. I use better body mechanics, being sure to stay low and use my legs more than my back. My back feels better.

Kim McCollum, CNA, Providence Benedictine
Nursing Center, Mt. Angel, OR

SUMMARY

A therapeutic transfer is an approach to assisting a person's mobility that maintains their functional abilities and is safe. This approach requires the caregiver to apply good body mechanics, attend to safety, and use clear communication. The appropriateness of a specific transfer method depends upon a person's functional abilities; the Transfer Progression Continuum identifies transfer methods which provide increasing caregiver assistance to balance a person's increasing dependence. The success of a therapeutic transfer program depends upon administrative support within the facility. In addition to the health and safety benefits for frail elders, attention to therapeutic transfers contributes to the spirit of teamwork and caregiver involvement in the provision of individualized care.

REFERENCES

Garg, A., & Owen, B. D. (1992). Reducing back stress of nursing personnel: An ergonomic intervention in a nursing home. *Ergonomics, 35,* 1353–1375.

Garg, A., Owen, B. D., & Carlson, B. (1992). An ergonomic evaluation of nursing assistant's job in a nursing home. *Ergonomics, 35,* 979–75.

Owen, B. D., Welden, N., & Kane, J. (1999). What are we teaching about lifting and transferring patients? *Research in Nursing and Health, 22,* 3–13.

CHAPTER 9

The Physical Environment of the Bathing Room

Margaret P. Calkins

Bathing does not occur in a void. It typically happens in a room which provides a visual, auditory, olfactory, thermal, and textural context. There are also spatial qualities of the room that can either cause problems, support independence, or support caregivers providing assistance. In general, space issues are the same regardless of the setting (home, assisted living, residential care, or nursing home), although some of the details may vary from setting to setting. Except when specifically noted, all suggestions in this chapter can be applied to all types of care settings. Suggestions will address both modification of existing bathing rooms and considerations for new construction. Since there is a separate chapter dealing with tub and shower equipment, this chapter concentrates on the environment around the tub or shower. Except as noted, the term "being bathed" refers to either taking a bath or a shower, and the term "bath room" refers to a room where a bath or shower is given. Finally, the focus here is on rooms specifically designed for bathing, and not bedrooms or other rooms in which sponge baths or other forms of cleansing might take place.

Because the environment is experienced primarily through our senses, this chapter is organized by sensory modality. The greatest emphasis is always given to how the person being bathed is experiencing the setting, with a secondary focus on the ways the environment can support the caregiver.

Visual Environment

Bath rooms in most long-term care settings are sterile, institutional, and frightening spaces filled with unfamiliar equipment—tubs with mechanical lifts or sides that open up and look like they might swallow you, chairs on wheels or gurneys with arms that look like construction cranes. There also may be soiled utility carts, scales, extra wheelchairs, and boxes of supplies through which the person must navigate. In homes, while there is likely to be less large equipment, the counters and ledges and other surfaces are often jammed with personal care products—three or four kinds of shampoo, several brushes and combs, a hair dryer, shoe-polishing kits, hair color kits—the list can go on and on. It's not surprising that the person who needs some assistance with bathing resists going in.

The first solution is to keep it simple. Find another location to store the extra equipment and supplies. If there is absolutely no other room available for the carts and lifts—or if they are necessary for bathing purposes—then build a partition to hide all that visually distracting stuff. You can keep it physically accessible, just not visually accessible. As a last resort, if there is no room to build a partition, hang a curtain so the storage part of the room is separate from the bathing part. If so, be creative; don't just use the standard, (i.e., dull) institutional shower curtain. There are a multitude of fire and moisture resistant fabrics that are much more decorative. And don't be chintzy about the size. Be sure there is ample fabric to hide everything (for more on this, see acoustics below).

At home, the same principle applies—reduce unnecessary visual clutter. You probably won't build a partition wall, but remove everything that is not essential. Consider adding an extra cupboard—in the bath room if there is room, or outside the door if the bath room is small. You want to simplify how the room looks but not make everyone else miserable because they cannot get to the things they want to use. If there is no room for a cabinet, give other bath room users their own basket or carrying case to hold personal toiletries.

Once you've eliminated the visual clutter from extra equipment and supplies, the next step is to make the room more visually pleasing. Think about where the person's eyes focus throughout the bathing process. It's best to get this from his/her perspective. If a wheelchair is used, have someone wheel you into the room. Consider wearing a pair of sunglasses smeared with a little petroleum jelly. This will mimic some of the visual changes that are common in elderly. Now, as you're being wheeled into the room, pay attention to where your eyes focus. What do you see when you first enter the room, as you get into the tub or shower, as you are being bathed, and when you are getting out and being dried? What is there to look at during each stage of the bath? For instance, individual supplies for each person are often kept in an open cabinet with cubbyholes and plastic baskets, marked with names on masking tape. While this is convenient, it looks more like a kindergarten storage area than a bath room. Get a cabinet with decorative doors, or paint a pretty pattern on a plain door, or as a last resort get a decorative curtain to make this prettier.

Do signs and notices about how to use different pieces of equipment constitute the only "art" in the room? If so, try to make them less conspicuous to the person being bathed. Laminate posters or prints to keep them dry in the moist atmosphere of the room, and hang them where the person is likely to see them. Add small decorative shelves with knickknacks such as shells, decorative bottles, pretty hand towels, or boxes for tissues. Pay particular attention to where the person is looking during the bath or shower. If they are reclined, could you put a print on the ceiling? If the tub control panel (which is often very institutional looking) is not part of the tub but hanging on the wall, see if the tub can be turned to give the bather a different view. Otherwise, cover the control panel with a curtain so it's not so visible. Consider replacing drab shower curtains with more decorative ones. In the shower, laminated photos may provide something interesting to look at. Some facilities even put up photos or drawings of the different steps in the bathing process, to cue the person to what will happen next.

Often the walls as well as the floor of bath rooms are tiled. While this is useful for cleaning, it is often not aesthetically appealing. Inexpensive, decorative stick-on tile covers are available at home or bed and bath stores and in many catalogues. Depending on the wall surface (drywall vs. tile vs. solid surface), it may be possible to add a decorative border. Ask a volunteer to stencil a pattern around the room. Consider placing these decorative touches at eye level, so they are easily visible to the person being bathed. Aquatic themes are often considered—beaches, fishes, dolphins, penguins, etc.

Another strategy that can help—both in downplaying institutional features and highlighting a residential feel—is the use of visual contrast. Many older people, and particularly people with dementia, have decreased contrast perception. Therefore, when there are necessary institutional features (such as signs or equipment), the more you can make them the same color as the background, the less they will be perceived. For residential features—such as art or knickknacks—you are adding to the environment; so make sure they stand out visually in the environment, by giving them a brighter color that contrasts with the background color of the walls.

Because bath rooms at home are often small, it is generally best to make the environment as simple as possible. We've already discussed eliminating extra personal care products. Another concern may include removing or covering mirrors, if they (as happens sometimes in dementia) are distracting or disturbing. Camouflage techniques include covering mirrors with laminated prints, or sticking the print on with a sticky-back Velcro™ tab (this allows the mirror to be used by others). If the mirror is on a metal back (like a medicine cabinet) you can purchase sticky-back magnet strips at a hardware store and attach these to the back of the print. If a mirror is flat against the wall, and the walls are covered with wallpaper, continue the wallpaper over the mirror.

Finally, lighting is very important in bath rooms. It needs to be sufficient—particularly near the tub and shower—so you can see that the person is getting clean. If the person being bathed is looking up (in a reclined position or lying prone on a bath gurney), be sure no lights shine directly into their eyes. Get into the tub or lie on the bath gurney and see what they are looking at. If you need to add lights, consider cove lighting, which bounces light off the ceiling (this is called indirect lighting), or wall sconces.

While it needs to be adequate, lighting should not be so bright that it feels overly clinical. Some people may actually be more comfortable in a room with softer lighting. Therefore, the best solution is to get the lights

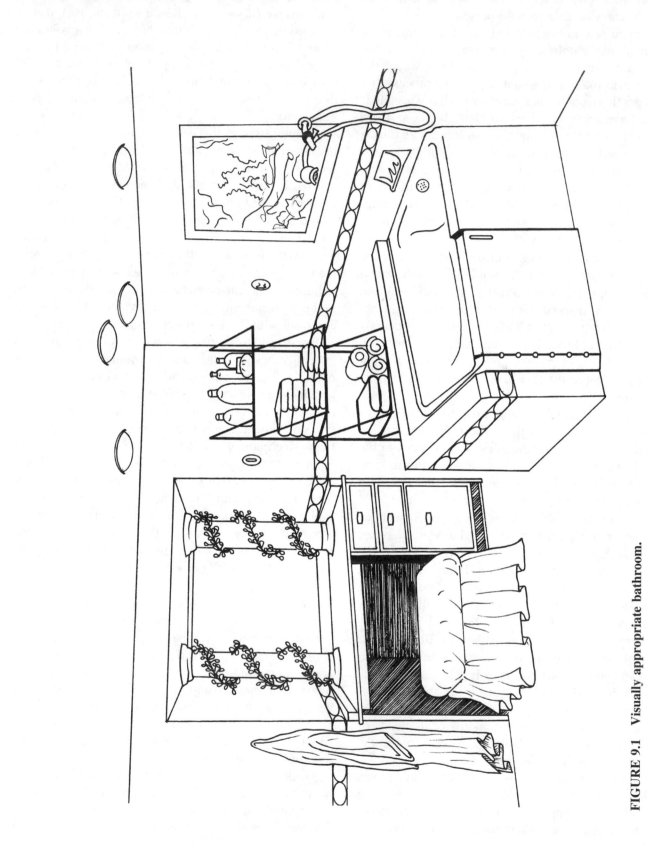

FIGURE 9.1 Visually appropriate bathroom.

Adapted from the Warren Barr Pavilion, designed by Studio One Designs.

on a rheostat so they can be individually adjusted for each person's preference. If this is not possible, see if some of the lights can be switched individually, so you can turn some, but not all, lights on. Also consider adding a table lamp, especially if there is a dressing table (see Spatial Environment). Finally, given that so much skin is exposed during bathing, it is important to have full spectrum lightbulbs because they make the skin a warm and healthier looking color.

Auditory Environment

Noise is distracting and can be agitating to persons being bathed. To reduce bath room noise, there are two basic techniques. The first is to stop the noise at its source. Thus, the first and foremost rule is never to bathe more than one person at a time—especially with people who do not particularly like bath time. Hearing the sounds from another tub or shower, and the people talking (often speaking in a loud voice to be heard over the noise of the water or the whirlpool pumps) can be very distracting and disturbing. The second rule for stopping noise at the source is to not let others walk into the bath room when someone is being bathed. This is why is it so important to try to get extra carts and stored equipment out of the bath room when possible. The sound of someone opening the door and coming in is enough to set some people off, fearing even more for their already compromised privacy.

The other basic technique to minimize noise is to add sound-absorbent materials. Sound bounces off tile and other solid surfaces and floors; so, to reduce this reverberation, add fabric-lined window and shower curtains. As a general rule of thumb, the fabric should be three to four times the width of the opening to have sufficient folds to maximize sound absorption. Another approach is to add water-resistant acoustic panels. These can be plain or decorative. The more walls (and ceiling) are covered by sound-absorbent tiles, the quieter the room. (See chapter appendix for suppliers of acoustic panels.)

Once negative noises and echoes are under control, you can consider the therapeutic benefits of adding positive sounds, such as music. A small collection of CDs that includes gospel, classical, new age, some oldies, and possibly country will suit almost anyone. Better yet, try to find a few tunes you can both sing along

to ("I'm gonna wash that man right out of my hair" from South Pacific comes to mind as especially appropriate).

Caregiver Wisdom

If they like music, I play what they like. It relaxes them to hear the music they like.

Mimi Leavenworth, Head CNA, Willametteview Convalescent Center, Portland, OR

Olfactory Environment

One doesn't generally think of the olfactory environment in relation to bathing, yet bath rooms are often characterized by lingering (or sometimes powerful) remnants of urine and excrement. Opening the door to a bath room with these odors will certainly not get the bath off to the right start.

The best way to eliminate these odors is not to let soiled clothing, sheets, or incontinence products sit in the bath room. This is an admirable goal, but not always feasible, especially in a home setting where a trip to the trash can out back after every change may not be realistic.

If odors are present, it is important to minimize them. There are two ways to do this. The first is to try to get at the source. Even if soiled products have been removed, they may leave a lingering odor in the hamper. Or if there has been an accident, the odor can linger in the seams and joints of the floor. To prevent lingering odors, clean these areas thoroughly and regularly with a strong disinfectant. If there are cracks in the floor, or between the floor and the baseboard of the wall, seal them (clear silicone available at hardware stores works well). The other method is to simply mask the odors by spraying with a room freshener or using plug-in fresheners. Long-term care settings may want to install deodorizers that spray a fine mist of air freshener into the bath room at regular intervals.

Once negative odors are minimized, you can consider adding positive aromas. An aroma therapy diffuser can be filled with a variety of calming essential oils, such as sweet marjoram, lavender, ylang-ylang, and clary sage. If this seems impractical, simply spray a little scented room freshener in the bath room a minute or so before bringing the person in. Recognize, however, that these sprays seldom last very long.

Scented bath oils can also be pleasing, although they often cannot be used in tubs with whirlpool mechanisms. Alternatively, a variety of scented body soaps may work well. Another approach is to apply a scented body oil or lotion after the bath.

Tactile Environment

As mentioned above, bath rooms are typically full of hard surfaces. This is important because of the moisture and the need to clean the area between baths. But it does not make for a very comfortable experience. When you think of being comfortable, you typically think of being surrounded by warm, soft materials.

Most people at home have either carpeting or a bath rug on the bath room floor. Tiles are cold and uncomfortable on the feet—try standing around naked and wet on a tile floor, and see how uncomfortable it is. While carpeting a bath room in a long-term care facility may be impractical, having something soft on the floor, like a (washable) rug, can make a big difference to the experience.

The other aspect of flooring that is important to consider is how slippery it is when wet. If installing a new floor, select a material with a high coefficient of friction (COF)—ideally above 80. There are also a number of coatings that can be used with existing floors to increase the COF. See the list of resources at the end of this chapter, or check on the World Wide Web, searching for nonslip flooring. (See chapter appendix for suppliers of nonslip flooring.)

For some people, there is nothing more wonderful than being wrapped in a warm towel or blanket. There are commercial towel warmers available which can make this aspect of bathing a much more luxuriant experience. (See chapter appendix for suppliers of towel warmers.)

Also, for people who do not particularly like being bathed, think about providing soft things they can hold, such as washcloths or personal sponges. When these have been in warm water, they not only give the hands something to hold, they serve to encourage the person to help with their own bathing.

When people are using showers, it is important to have stable grab bars to hold for balance. For many years, we have relied on stainless steel grab bars, which are aesthetically unappealing and often cold and hard to the touch. Now there are a variety of powder-coated grab bars that come in decorative colors and have a nonslip grip (which is crucial). The location of grab bars in institutional settings is generally regulated by the Americans with Disabilities Act (ADA), although research suggests that these are not always the most useful locations for elderly individuals. The ADA regulations require a grab bar to the side of the toilet and behind the tank, mounted level to the floor, 33–36 inches above the floor. Many older adults find a side bar angled at approximately 45 degrees is better, because elderly individuals tend to pull themselves up, rather than push down on a bar. There are also bars that can swing away or fold up, making it easier for a caregiver to provide assistance, should it be needed. In the tub or shower, there should be horizontal grab bars on all walls, 33–36 inches above the floor. Many institutional tubs come with grab bars preinstalled. While not required by the ADA, a 24-inch vertical bar at the point of entry into the shower/tub is also useful. All grab bars should be 1 1/2 inches in diameter, and 1 1/2 inches from the wall. There is an excellent website for home modifications for bath rooms, listed in the resource list at the end of this chapter. (See chapter appendix for suppliers of grab bars.)

The temperature of the room is critically important to the comfort of the person being bathed. Older people are highly sensitive to drafts and are easily chilled. Anyone taking a shower is likely to have a significant amount of exposed, wet skin, which can quickly feel cold. Also, many of the tubs available on the market only cover the bather from the waist down, leaving the upper portion of the body wet and exposed to drafts and chills. Thus, every bath room should be equipped with an extra source of heat. If the caregiver is overly warm, almost to the point of sweating, the temperature is probably about right for the older person being bathed. Common sources of heat include heat lamps or radiant heat panels. Be sure the heat source is not a potential fire or electrocution hazard. No products that include exposed heating elements should be placed in a bath room. Also, all heating elements should be mounted permanently to the wall or ceiling, to avoid the possibility of coming in contact with water.

Caregiver Wisdom

I make sure the room is warm. If there's a heater in the room, I turn it up. If there is no heater, I let the water run before I bring the person in so it feels steamy and warm when we enter.

Mimi Leavenworth, Head CNA, Willametteview
Convalescent Center, Portland, OR

Finally, while not necessarily apparent to the person being bathed, it is extremely helpful to have at least one floor drain in all bath rooms. This helps deal efficiently with excess water should the shower or tub overflow. It also makes cleaning the room much easier.

Spatial Environment

There is much debate about whether bath rooms should be spacious (to provide room for caregivers and equipment) or cozy (to avoid that "institutional" feel). The answer, ideally, is both. And fortunately, these issues are not mutually exclusive.

Recognizing that many people need assistive devices (such as a wheelchair, walker, or lift), all bath rooms should provide sufficient space for use of these appliances. The standard five-foot turning radius specified by the Americans with Disabilities Act was not based on the needs of a physically frail older population with limited upper body strength. Relatively few older individuals using wheelchairs can turn around in a 5-foot space with less than five or six turning points. A 7-foot radius is better. The ideal amount of space depends on the type of bathing equipment (bath vs. tub), other equipment (lifts, toilet, sink, vanity, etc.) and their location within the room. The best way to determine if there is enough room (particularly if you are considering new construction or major renovations) is to lay out the space and try it out. This process can be as simple as putting tape on the floor to designate the walls and fixtures, or laying folding tables on their side to designate walls. Ask a typical user to try out the space to see how well it works. Be sure to include a caregiver in the space if the person being bathed needs assistance.

Other amenities within the room are important to how the space feels. As mentioned previously, the décor of bath rooms is often cold and sterile. Adding color, wallpaper, borders, and visually interesting art or knick-knacks can easily change the character. Most people would probably prefer to undress and dress in the bath room instead of doing so in their bedroom and being wheeled down the hallway in a sheet. Therefore, be sure that there are places to hang fresh clothes (such as a few decorative hooks on the wall) and to put away soiled clothes (i.e., a laundry hamper). For many people, bathing is associated with grooming, so having a small dressing table with a good mirror and warm lighting can also be helpful.

Conclusions

In long-term care settings, the bath room is one of the strongest remnants of the old institutional model, where the goals of efficiency and utility still reign supreme over the psychological and emotional comfort of the person being bathed. But this can, and indeed must, change to reflect our changing cultural values about long-term care. If the priorities in long-term care are to recognize and support the cognitive, emotional, psychological, and spiritual needs of individuals as well as their physical needs, then all spaces need to reflect these goals. This is especially true for spaces where the most personal care—such as bathing—is provided. How a facility manages the minutia of life, such as the bathing process, including how bath rooms are designed and decorated, can speak volumes about the quality of a care setting.

REFERENCES

Alzheimer's List Serve. (2000). [On-line]. Available: alzheimer@wubios.wustl.edu

Kearney, D. (1992). *The New ADA: Compliance and Costs.* Kingston, MA: Construction Publishers & Consultants.

Sloane, P., Honn, V., Dwyer, S., Wieselquist, J., Cain, C., & Meyers, S. (1995). Bathing the Alzheimer's patient in long-term care: Results and recommendations from three studies. *American Journal of Alzheimer's Disease, 10*(4), 3–12.

Warner, M. (1999). *Alzheimer's proofing your home.* West Lafayette, IN: Purdue University Press.

Web-site for home modifications to bath rooms: http://www.intersource.com/~srnet/MCSN_Websites/homemod/HMbathgb.html or search for "grab bars" on the Web.

APPENDIX

Selected Products and Manufacturers

PRODUCT	PURPOSE	MANUFACTURERS
Grab Bars	Provide additional support when using toilet, getting out of tub, or in the shower.	Bobrick 518-877-7444 U.S. Builder Supply 877-378-5625 www.usbuildersupply.com Wholesale Bath 6700 Barnes Settlement Road Northport, AL 35473 888-748-5732 www.wholesalebath.com Wingits Innovations 181 W. Clay Ave. Roselle Park, NJ 07204 877-894-6448 www.wingits.com (special bolts that allow installation of grab bars through simple drywall) Sarff Systems Inc. 3519 N. Eden, Suite B Spokane, WA 99216 877-398-3635 www.extendahand.com www.grabbars.com Elcoma 1929 36th St. N.E. Canton, OH 44705 800-352-6625 www.elcoma.com TSM Box 60262 Los Angeles, CA 90060 800-225-5876 www.TSM.com
Acoustic Panels	Reduce noise reverberation and echoes	Illbruck Acoustic Panels 3800 Washington Ave N Minn. MN 55412 800-225-1920 Conwed Designscape 1205 Worden Ave. East Ladysmith, WI 54848 800-932-2383

Selected Products and Manufacturers

PRODUCT	PURPOSE	MANUFACTURERS
Half-height Shower Curtains	Help keep the caregiver dry when providing assistance to someone showering	Silcraft Corporation 528 Hughes Drive Traverse City, MI 49683 800-678-7100
Flooring	Nonslip flooring	Safe Step Non-slip Inc. 29453 Mulholland Hwy. Box 991 Agoura Hills, CA 91376 800-865-0260 www.safestepnon-slip.com Secure Step International, Inc. 800-288-4213 www.securestep.com Sure Foot Maintenance Compounds 1633 Flat Rd. RR1 Dacre Ontario Canada K0J 1N0 613-649-2000 www.surefoot.bc.ca M.L. Thornton Enterprises 1014 Hopper Ave. Suite 253 Santa Rosa, CA 95493 707-525-0770 www.getagrip-nonslip.com Trend Coatings 1805 Porter Lake Rd. Suite 107 Sarasota, FL 34233 800-632-2063 www.quarztex.com
Towel Warmer	Keeps several towels warm and ready to use	Imperial Surgical Ltd. 189 Danison St. Markham Ontario Canada L3R 1B5 905-470-6060

CHAPTER 10

Equipment and Supplies

Philip D. Sloane and Leanne E. Carnes

Most people enjoy a good bath or shower. They love to soak in a deep tub of fragrant bubbles. They relish the gentle massage of warm spray on their neck, shoulders, and back. They like nothing better than to lean back, close their eyes, and feel Jacuzzi jets fizz against naked skin. And, when the bath is over, there's the delicious feeling of wrapping one's tingling body in luxurious terrycloth. These and other pleasures of bathing depend on proper equipment and supplies. Indeed, the products make or break the experience; the products provide the comfort, luxury, and sensuality.

Baths have a practical function, too. They remove dirt, sweat, and debris from the body, improving one's appearance. They kill and remove unwanted bacteria, thereby preventing infection. And they remove unwanted odors, rendering the individual more socially acceptable. These functions depend on bathing equipment, supplies, and instruction and/or supervision by a caregiver(s).

As is noted elsewhere in this book, bathing is often not pleasurable for a person with Alzheimer's disease or a related dementia. A variety of caregiving strategies described elsewhere in this book provide the cornerstone of effective bathing for persons with these diseases. However, equipment and supplies have an important role, as well. For persons with dementia, just as for the general public, choosing the right equipment and supplies can make the difference between a pleasurable, effective bath and an unpleasant, ineffective one.

This chapter discusses the wide range of bathing equipment and supplies that are available to care providers of persons with dementia. It focuses on institutional settings such as nursing homes and assisted living; however, much of the information is also relevant to family caregivers. Equipment related to showers, tub baths,

and bed baths is described. A discussion of accessories and supplies that can be helpful in specific situations is also included. Because individual products and brand names often change rapidly, the chapter concentrates on general principles and types of equipment, rather than on specific products.

Showers

Showering is the most common bathing method used by U.S. adults, including persons in long-term care. Compared with a tub bath, the shower is faster, uses less water, provides more thorough rinsing, and allows for washing the body in parts. It is not as good as the bath for removing dried, crusted, or caked material from the skin. It is also less safe for persons with significant balance problems or frequent falls. Furthermore, caregiver assistance is often difficult to provide in a traditional shower. For this reason, open shower areas and portable nozzles are often used in long-term care, but this procedure often makes the bather chilly. So, while showers are common and have many advantages, they also present challenges, especially in the care of persons with dementia.

Making the Shower Practical for Bathers and Staff

The shower must be accessible. Ideally, the bather should be able to walk or be rolled into the shower as easily as into a room, and caregiver access should be easy. There should be a smooth transition of floor surface as you enter the shower area. In combination shower-tubs, where a smooth floor transition is not possible, the bather must either be capable of stepping over the tub wall or have another means of getting into the shower (see Bathtubs section). Also, shower-tubs should use a shower curtain or a hinged door instead of a sliding door, because sliding doors always block half of the doorway, thereby limiting access.

The shower area must foster easy bathing. Products for cleaning the bather must be close at hand; if the bather is behaviorally disruptive or physically unable, they should be available to the caregiver but out of reach for the bather. The showerhead must be in a position where the caregiver can access it without the showerhead or hose dragging across the bather. Towels and extra washcloths must also be close at hand to make the bath as thorough and quick as possible.

The shower should be strategically placed within the bathing room. It should be beyond visual range of the door so that: 1) the way out is not seen, and 2) privacy will not be lost if the door into the bathing area is accidentally opened.

There should be a place for the bather to sit in the shower. This will cut down on fatigue and give the bather a sense of security. Some shower setups even allow the bather to lie down. This can be accomplished by including a built-in seat, a removable shower chair (Figures 10.1 and 10.2) or a shower gurney (described later in this section); however, tub or in-room bathing is often preferred to a shower for persons who are unable to sit or stand safely.

Safety Issues in Showers

Safety issues vary according to the shower's layout and accessories. Floors in a shower are wet and can be slippery; so nonslip flooring is essential. If a shower chair is used, the right torque and angle may cause it to topple. To avoid this, some chairs can be locked into the walls of the shower. Other chairs have wheels that lock and nonslip surfaces on the bottom of the chair.

Hot water burns may also occur in the shower. Antiscalding devices are highly recommended to alleviate this problem. There are two types: One attaches to the water heater; the other is built into the tub or shower. Both are designed to prevent water temperatures from getting too hot. The water in a water heater with an antiscalding device should be set to 125–130° Fahrenheit and between 104–106° for tubs and showers.

Many people prefer to stand in the shower, because it gives them a sense of normality and control. Others are asked to stand, because that position is excellent

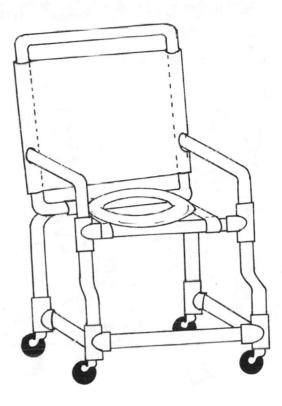

FIGURE 10.1   Shower chair with toilet seat.

for washing the genitals and anal area. To prevent falls among standing bathers, grab bars need to be easy to find, easy to grip, and easy to reach by people of varying heights (when going from sitting to standing). They must always be present in locations where a bather is likely to transfer or stand up from a chair.

Cleaning and Maintaining Shower Areas

Showers must be disinfected after every bath, but few come with disinfecting systems. The walls, floor, and grab bars are all parts of the shower that need to be cleaned after every bath. A grooved tile surface is more difficult and time consuming to disinfect than a smooth fiberglass surface.

The drain needs special attention. The drain must be cleared of all residues from the previous shower. A second drain catch can be placed under the first drain catch to prevent larger debris from going into the pipes. This will help prevent the pipes from being clogged, and water resurfacing from inside the drain.

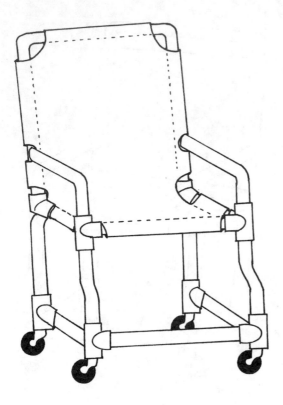

FIGURE 10.2 Shower chair with solid seat.

Available Products

Custom (or general) residential shower stalls are the shower stalls found in a personal residence. They usually consist of three plastic or tile walls, a door, and an elevated drain platform (the floor slopes to a central drain). These types of showers have the option of adding or installing grab bars, seats, and a ramp. The door can be hinged or sliding, or it can be removed and replaced with a curtain.

Roll-in Showers have a barrier-free entrance. A gradual ramp leads up to the shower entrance and the shower base slopes down to a central drain. The entrance to most of these shower stalls is wide enough for wheelchair passage. They come with the option of a door or a shower curtain. Examples of roll-in showers include Model #5530 (Diversified Fiberglass Fabrications) and VBF6030 BASE (Venco).

A *seated shower* looks like a tub but is not meant to hold water. Seated showers come with a built-in seat, a handheld showerhead, and a door. They may have the option of the seat sliding in and out of the tub to

help ease in transfer. An example of a seated shower is the Prelude (Arjo).

A *shower-tub* is the combination of a bathtub and a shower. The bather has the option of taking a shower or a bath. These come with the option to install an attached or unattached bath seat, transfer bench, grab bars, and handheld showerhead. There is also the option of a sliding door or shower curtain. Some of these shower-tubs include Model 45R/LF (National Bathing Products), V6032HTS (Venco), and Aqua Glass Acrylic Bath (Aqua Glass).

Shower Accessories

Shower accessories are products that can be added or built into the shower. Shower accessories are listed and described in Table 10.1. General bathing supplies, which are useful in showers, tub baths, or bed baths, are listed and described in Table 10.2.

Caregiver Wisdom

You have to choose the right shower chair. If the one you have doesn't fit the person, you adapt it. You can pad the seat with washcloths to make it softer. You can use a kid's padded potty seat insert available at stores for about $10.00 to make the hole smaller and the seat more comfortable.

Kathy House, CNA, Fairlawn Good Samaritan
Health Center, Gresham, OR

Bathtubs

A tub bath is traditionally considered the most relaxing and luxurious method of bathing. Oils, bubbles, and other products have been developed for tub bathing that can add to this feeling of luxury. The tub bath also has the advantage of allowing the bather to soak, thereby loosening stubborn dirt and debris and relieving stiffness in muscles and joints. Also, it is safer and more comfortable for persons with mobility problems because they do not have to support their posture. Transfers can be hazardous, however, and must be done with care (see chapter 8). The traditional bathtub is low and located in the corner of a room. This makes caregiver access difficult. However, a number of specialized tubs and tub products can make tub use easier when assis-

TABLE 10.1 Shower Accessories

Accessory	Description and Purpose	Options	Comments	Examples of Manufacturers
Shower Chair	Lightweight chair with commode seat and mesh back. Allows the resident to sit during the shower.	Plastic pipe or metal. With/without wheels. Variation in width. Extended foot rest.	Not comfortable for some residents Some residents fall through the hole in the seat.	Briggs PVC Pipe Co. ASI
Soft Seat Shower Chair	Similar to the regular shower chair, but the seat is cushioned. Allows for added comfort in the shower.	Padded plastic pipe or metal. With/without wheels. Variation in width. Extended foot rest.	Some residents feel as if they are sliding through the hole in the seat.	Briggs PVC Pipe Co. ASI
Shower Gurney or Trolley	Horizontal shower chair with side barriers and a drain. Allows the resident to lay down during the shower.	Locking wheels. Plastic pipe or metal with mesh, foam bed or molded plastic. Attachable draining tube. Removable or fold down sides. Varies in length and width.	Reported to be scary and unfamiliar to the residents. Big and hard to store. Mesh does not allow all the debris to pass through it.	Conva quip Universal
Poncho	Outer cover to aid in heat retention during the shower.	Plastic or water-resistant fabric. Hood, or no hood. Many colors.	Expensive for what it is, as a towel may work just as well.	Briggs
Handheld Showerhead	Mobile showerhead with pressure control. Allows for more controlled rinsing.	Pause and/or on/off controls on the head. White or chrome. Metal or Plastic extension tube.	Needs to have a pressure control gauge.	Briggs GAMCO Activated, Inc. Access with Ease Sears Home HealthCare Catalogue
Antiscald Device	Monitors the hot water temperature to prevent burns	Available as specialized showerhead or an insert into an existing showerhead	A necessity in the bathing room.	Memry Corporation Accent on Living Keeney Brookstone Joan Cook

tance is needed. Other disadvantages include difficulty reaching the genital area and the possibility that an incontinent person will lose control while in the tub.

Considerations in Selecting a Tub

The first thing to consider when selecting a tub is who will be using the tub. The "who" refers to both the caregiver(s) and the person(s) receiving the bath. Following are some questions and issues to address in choosing a specific bathtub:

- *How accessible is the tub to bathers and caregivers?*

Getting into and out of the tub should be easy for the bather. If the bather has mobility or balance problems, tub entry and exit can be accomplished by means of caregiver assistance, a lift, a door built into the tub, or by using a transfer bench or chair.

A lift usually requires one person to operate, thus increasing the bather's privacy. The lift also helps prevent caregiver injuries. On the down

TABLE 10.2 General Bathing Supplies

General bathing supplies are products that may be used in any bathing solution, according to the needs of the bather. These produces are made and/or supplied by many companies such as Access One, ASI, Briggs, Colgate, GAMCO, Gillette, MediSkin, and Tubular Specialties Mfg.

Product	Purpose	Description of Product	Options
No-rinse soap/Cleaner	To clean skin without water.	A liquid product that is applied to the skin to remove dirt and odor.	Gel Foam Lotion Solution
Liquid Soap	To clean skin without overdrying.	A liquid product that is applied to wet skin and then rinsed off to remove dirt and odor.	Fragrance Nonlathering
Liquid Lotion Soap	Skin conditioning and cleansing in one.	A liquid product that cleans and moisturizes the skin.	Rinseable No-rinse
Bar Soap	To clean the skin.	Traditional method of cleaning the skin, needs water to apply and remove.	Fragrance Moisturizer Texture
Incontinent cleanser/ Deodorizer	For cleaning perineum area between baths.	Product that when applied cleans and disinfects; does not require water to rinse.	Gel Foam Liquid Liquid spray Moisturizer
Body Wash and Shampoo	For cleaning entire body from head to toe.	A combined product used to clean the body, face, and hair.	Moisturized Fragrance Gel No-rinse
Shampoo	To clean hair.	Traditional method of cleaning the hair; requires water to apply and remove.	Fragrance Hair type Dandruff
Shampoo + Conditioner	Hair moisturizing and cleaning in one.	A product that cleans and moisturizes the hair.	Rinseable No-rinse Fragrance
Conditioner	To moisturize hair.	Traditional method of moisturizing the hair.	Rinseable No-rinse Fragrance
Dandruff shampoo	To clean hair and aid in the cessation of dandruff.	A shampoo product; requires water to rinse.	Prescription Nonprescription
Lotion	Moisturize skin.	Traditional method to moisturize the skin.	Fragrance Thickness
Washcloth	Aid in lathering/agitation of cleansing products. Remove dead skin cells	A small cloth used for spreading and agitating cleansing products.	Woven Nonwoven Colors
Towel	Dry the resident. Keep resident warm.	Large absorbent cloth.	Woven Nonwoven Colors
Disposable Washcloths	Decrease the spread of contaminants.	One-time-use washcloths for cleaning.	Prepackaged with cleanser Size
Examination Gloves	Prevent disease transmission.	Protective barrier between caregiver and resident.	Latex Vinyl

TABLE 10.2 (continued)

Product	Purpose	Description of product	Options
Deodorant	Prevent body odor.	Product applied to underarms to prevent odors.	Stick Roll-on Spray
Tooth Swab	Oral cleaning scrubber.	A soft tip on a stick to clean teeth.	Foam tip Rubber tip Fiber tip
Toothpaste	Clean teeth.	Oral cleaner.	Tarter control Fluoride Gel/paste
Toothbrush	Lather/agitate oral cleaner.	Oral cleaning utensil.	Electric Manual
Shaving Cream	Prevent cuts during shaving. Moisturize face.	Topical product applied to face for shaving.	Gel Foam Cream
Toe Washer	Wash between toes.	A thin stick with a scrubber on the end.	Foam tip Rubber tip Fiber tip
Incontinent Commode Bath	To wash perineum area between baths using soap and water without giving the person a full bath.	A toilet seat attachment that rinses the soiled area.	Adjustable water pressure
Perineum Wash	Cleans and disinfects perineum area. Can be used during and between baths.	Cleansing product for very soiled areas.	Rinse No-rinse Gel Liquid Foam Moisturizer
Disinfectant Cleaner	Clean and disinfect the bathing area.	Disinfectant type cleaner used for infection control after every bath.	Scrub-free Liquid Foam

side, the lift also takes training and tends to be tedious to set up and operate. Also, it can be a frightening experience for the bather, especially persons with dementia. Mechanical lifts are often noisy, and the noise and movement can be confusing or threatening. Some facilities do not use tubs at all with demented residents because, in their experience, lift use has caused violent outbursts. However, lift systems that do not raise the bather high in the air can reduce this problem.

One nonlift transfer system is a door built into the tub. The doors allow the bather to walk into or be guided into the tub. The major drawback is that the bather then needs to sit in the tub while it fills, and the fill time may be quite long. Some bathers welcome the break, however, as it allows them to settle down. Bathers will be warmer during tub filling if their shoulders are covered with a towel or blanket. A more difficult problem with tub doors is that they tend to break, leak, or seal incorrectly over time.

Transfer benches and chairs provide another nonlift solution (Figure 10.3). The tub can be filled prior to the bather getting into the tub. Transfer benches can help promote bather independence by allowing more control in entering the tub. They should generally be used with supervision, however, to decrease falls and bather frustration. For bathers with severe mobility problems or who resist care, the process of assisting the bather using a transfer bench can be hard on the caregiver's back.

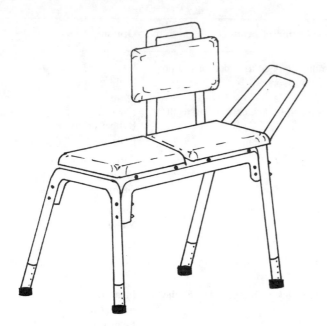

FIGURE 10.3   Transfer bench.

Caregiver access is another important issue in tub selection. Some tubs are built high enough so that caregivers do not need to bend. Others have a built-in motor that allows them to be raised and lowered. Others are low and require caregivers to bend. In such situations, caregivers can have bathers sit in a chair or seat in the tub, or they can themselves sit on low chairs or stools to prevent long periods of bending.

- *How safe is the tub?*
Safety issues in a tub bathing area are many. One is the risk of staff injury from bending over or transferring an impaired bather. Another is the risk of bather injury due to encountering hard or sharp surfaces, or to accidental slips or falls. These risks can be minimized through proper equipment selection and staff training. Safety equipment includes ergonomically designed tubs, pressure controls on water outlets, antiscald temperature controls, properly placed grab bars, a handheld shower head with a pause or on/off control on the head, and nonslip surfaces.

- *How easy is the tub to keep clean?*
A multiple-user tub must be disinfected after every bath; this is both a legal and a hygienic requirement. The disinfecting system can be a part of the tub or a completely different device(s).

Some tubs (especially those with jet systems) come with a built-in disinfecting system. Other bathtubs have to be manually disinfected. Most disinfecting systems have safety controls that prevent use in unauthorized times or when the system is malfunctioning. In either case, the tub must be easy to clean. Easy-to-clean, nonporous surfaces are a common feature of most tubs.

- *How effective is the tub in cleaning stool, urine, and debris from private areas?*
In order to maintain hygiene, a tub must allow easy access to every part of the bather. If the bather is sitting, there must be a way to clean underneath. For this purpose different types of seats can be used. There are mesh seats and seats with a hole in the base. There are also strategically placed grab bars so that the person can pull or assist in pulling to one side and then the other, so that the underside can be reached and cleaned. Some tubs provide jets or ultrasonic devices which, while not directly providing caregiver access, can help loosen debris from private areas.

Available Products

There are many products available when it comes to a bathtub and bathtub accessories. Because so many exist, and new ones appear frequently, this section will provide an overview of the basic types available, with examples of each.

There are four major tub types: 1) residential tubs, 2) water agitation tubs, 3) tubs with a door, and 4) bathing tables. The first type is a general tub; the latter three types are specialized tubs.

Residential tubs allow for a more homelike atmosphere. These are the tubs that we may have in our private homes. Such tubs can be adapted for special populations with the addition of certain accessories. Grab bars and seats can be added. Nonslip surfaces can be laid down. Handheld showerheads and antiscald temperature controls can be installed. The major benefits of these tubs are familiarity and price. The downside is that they may not be appropriate, and may even be dangerous, for certain populations. A bather who cannot stand or sit without assistance may find him/herself in danger of slips, falls, or even possibly drowning if left unattended. Also, bathers who resist care cannot be safely managed in a tub that does not have access from all sides; so, residential tubs that are recessed against a wall are not suitable for such persons. Examples of residential tub manufacturers include National Bathing Products and Vencor.

Specialized tubs allow for different and sometimes very specific options for special populations. Among the features available in specialized tubs are entry doors, integrated lifts, bedside attachments, whirlpool jets, hydro sound, movable/immovable seating, built-in grips and/or bars, and self-contained disinfecting systems. These tubs vary in price and may be unnecessary for some populations. For example, a person who is self-reliant would not benefit from a specialized tub and can use the less expensive general tub. Also, no specialized tub is perfect for more than a minority of persons with dementia; therefore, it is impossible to find a single tub that works for all.

Water agitation tubs have either whirlpool or hydro sound systems. Water agitation is used as a massage aid and to loosen debris. It is useful for bathers who are very stiff and need assistance in loosening their joints. There are two types of water agitation systems:

- Whirlpool systems have jets that circulate the water. The jets often come with pressure control.
- Hydro sound is water agitation without jets. The water is agitated by the use of ultrasonic waves. This often comes with frequency control.

Water agitation tubs vary in length and shape. Some come with a lift attached; others have a door. Some accommodate the seated position; in others the bather is lying down. Some come with a built-in seat, some supply a removable seat and others don't have any seat options. Examples of manufacturers of water agitation tubs include Arjo and Ferno.

Tubs with a door attempt to alleviate the need for a lift. The doors on such tubs allow the bather to get in and out of the tub with little to no assistance. The door is designed to have a watertight seal so the tub can be filled without leaking. These tubs may come with water agitation systems and/or disinfecting and skin-care systems. They also come in a variety of lengths and widths. Examples of such manufacturers include Arjo, Ferno, Silcraft, American Standard, BathEase, and Technically Unique.

A bathing table is a type of tub that is mainly used for severely disabled bathers. The table is an elevated flat surface with at least one drain and raised sides or railings. It can be assembled next to the bather's bed if there is a place to drain the water; however, it is used mostly in bathing areas. The bathing table allows the bather to get a shower while remaining horizontal. The tables come in a variety of different surfaces such as mesh cot, molded plastic, or nonporous fiberglass. Examples of bathing tables include Diversified Fiberglass, Bed Bather, and Arjo.

Tub Accessories

Tub accessories are the additional tools used in bath giving. These range from washcloths to independent lifts to types of soaps. Table 10.3 covers accessories exclusive to the bathtub. A tub insert (Figure 10.4) is an accessory that covers the tub completely to make the bottom of the tub higher and less deep. Other supplies that can be helpful in tub bathing are presented in Table 10.2.

Bed Bathing

Bed bathing provides an effective method of getting persons clean who have severe mobility problems or who fear and dislike tub baths and showers. It is valuable as an alternative for people who become upset or agitated during traditional baths. The bed bath has also been reported to be a very quick method of cleaning, especially when materials are organized in advance or prepackaged. Cleanliness will improve if the person tolerates a bed bath better than other methods, or if bed bathing increases the frequency of cleaning. Dry skin may improve with bed bathing, too, especially when a wet towel is applied to the skin for several minutes and lotion is applied immediately after drying. Bed baths

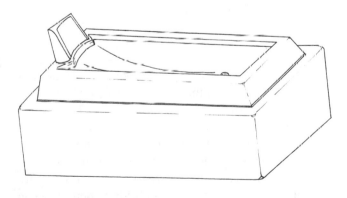

FIGURE 10.4   Tub insert.

TABLE 10.3 Bathtub Accessories

Accessory	Description and Purpose	Options	Comments	Examples of Manufacturers
Bath Seat	Small, lightweight plastic (usually), molded, drainage holes, easy-to-grip handles. Allows resident to bathe without getting down into the tub.	Seat back Leveling system	Resident gets cold out of the water	Rubbermaid Invacare Briggs
Bath Chair	Similar to Bath Seat but with a larger surface for sitting and a greater weight capacity. Allows resident to bathe without getting down inside the tub.	Seat back Leveling system	Resident gets cold out of the water Hard to store Takes up a lot of space	Rubbermaid Invacare Briggs
Transfer Bench	Slip resistant, molded, with right/left handles, drainage holes. Allows for an easier transfer to inside the tub.	Seat back Commode seat Commode pail Adjustable handles	Transfer may be hard on caregiver's back	Rubbermaid Briggs Inovated Products Unlimited
Transfer Board	Small, portable, easy to set/install, molded, drainage holes. Allows for an easier transfer to inside the tub.	Right/left handles Rubber or other nonslip bottom to grip and protect the tub Different lengths and widths	Tends to slide off bathtub side walls too much	Invacare Rubbermaid
Rails and Grips	Place on walls or on the side of the tub. Gives the resident something to hold on to for support and security.	Different shapes and angles for different gripping areas Grips with suction cups for individual bather placement Rubber or textured grips Adjustable and/or rubber-lined clamps Different thickness	Need to be anchored well onto the wall and into a supporting structure in the wall	Rubbermaid Briggs
Bath Mats	Rubber, carpeted or cloth surfaces that aide in slip proofing. Gives resident and caregiver security in stepping.	Rubber backing or suction cups to hold in place Variety of colors and textures	Mildew quickly if not cleaned often and/or are left wet	Invacare Linens and Things Rubbermaid
Tub Inserts	Lining that fits into most tubs without modification. Cushioned nonporous surface. Allows residents to bathe laying down.	Elevated end with wide transfer area Built-in seat	Hard to clean Too large to store easily	Diversified Fiberglass Fabrications

also minimize cross contamination because all materials are only used once and then are discarded or laundered.

One reported disadvantage of bed baths is that they may require greater attention and time than traditional showers or tub baths. However, if tub or shower disinfection and bather transport are factored in, bed baths may be faster than other methods. They do require constant temperature control and adjustment to keep the water warm enough. Basins of water have a tendency to spill and to require water changes when bathing very soiled areas, resulting in a lot of cleanup time at the end. The other limitation of bed bathing is that rinsing may be incomplete, leading to skin irritation.

Types of Bed Baths

There are three types of bed baths: the sponge bath, the towel bath (or bath in a bag), and the inflatable bed bathtub.

TABLE 10.4   Three Methods of Conducting a Bed Bath

	Type of Bath		
	Bag-prepackaged	**Sponge**	**Inflatable Tub**
Step 1	Microwave the entire package for 30 seconds or until warm. Do not overheat.	Fill a clean basin with warm water. Add soap and place on cart. Fill a second basin with warm water and place on cart.	Roll resident to one side.
Step 2	Open the package. Follow facility protocol on the order of areas cleaned.	Place 8–10 clean washcloths and 8–10 clean towels on the cart.	Place tub edge under resident and tub base where resident was lying.
Step 3	Use a different cloth for each of these body areas: 1) face neck and chest, 2) right arm/axilla, 3) left arm/axilla, 4) perineum, 5) right leg, 6) left leg, 7) back, 8) buttocks.	Clean the resident with the soapy water.	Roll resident back into original place (tub underneath).
Step 4	Discard cloths. *Do not reuse	Rinse and dry the resident with the nonsoapy water.	Make sure drain is not blocked. Fill tub to comfort of resident.
Step 5		Wash or discard the towels, washcloths and basins.	Bathe resident as if in bathtub.
Step 6		Clean any spills left in the room.	Drain bathtub (there is a hose attached to the drain hole for water to leave. Make sure the hose is draining into something that can hold all the water in the tub.
Step 7			Cover top of resident with towels for warmth. Deflate tub.
Step 8			Roll resident on his/her side and remove deflated tub. Dry resident. Disinfect tub according to protocol.

The sponge bath is a bath given with a basin full of soapy water and a sponge or washcloth. After a body area is washed, it is rinsed with a sponge and clean water, and then towel dried.

There are two types of *bag baths*. One is a commercial product that can be purchased with the cleaning agents and towels already inside a microwaveable bag. In the other type, the towel bath, the caregiver mixes the towels or cloths with the cleaning agents in a bag (in-house packaging). Prior to the bath, the soap and towels are mixed with hot water. Examples of prepackaged bag baths are the Bag Bath (Incline Technologies, Inc.) and the Comfort Bath (Sage Products, Inc.). For a description of a towel bath, see chapter 4.

The inflatable tub is a full-length bathtub made for bathing people in their bed. With the inflatable bathtub, the bather is rolled to one side while the tub is placed underneath; then the bather is rolled into place in the tub. Next, the tub is inflated using a mechanical pump or wet/dry vacuum, and filled with water to the comfort of the bather. Manufacturers of inflatable tubs include Invacare and Disability Products, Inc. For step-by-step instructions on bed bathing procedures, see Table 10.4.

Bed-Bath Accessories

Most bed-bath accessories are general products listed in Table 10.2. A few specialized bed-bath accessories exist. These include an inflatable bathtub, inflatable head basin, head cradle and bath blankets/sheets. The inflatable bathtub is designed to facilitate a bath in the bed. The head basin is used to wash the bather's hair in bed. It is typically inflated and slid under the head; a notch on one of the sides cradles the bather's neck.

TABLE 10.5 Level of Proper Assistive Devices

Independence Level	Abilities	Need	Product Example
Needs some stability support	Gets into and out of shower or tub without assistance	Slip resistant floor surface	Bath mat
Needs continual support while standing	Gets into and out of shower or bath with very little assistance	An easily accessible means of support	Grab bars, rails, and handles
Must sit for duration of the bathing process	Gets into and out of the shower or bath with guiding assistance	A sturdy place to sit	Stool
Needs back support and a place to sit during the bathing process	Needs assistance to sit in the tub or shower	A place to sit with back support	Chair
Cannot step into bathtub	Needs full assistance getting into and out of bath	Seated transfer into the tub	Bath board
Needs transfer and body support	Needs assistance getting into and out of tub and needs assistance sitting in the tub	Back support and a seated transfer into the tub	Transfer bench
Needs full transfer and body support	Can wash parts of self with prompting	Full body support, a place to sit and full bathing assistance	Lift

It drains by way of a tube in the base. The head cradle holds the same purpose as the inflatable basin; only the water is channeled off to the side for draining. And finally, bath blankets and sheets are useful; these are large towels that may or may not be woven. Blankets and sheets differ from each other in thickness and weight. They are used to help keep the bather warm, comfortable, and dry.

Conclusion

Proper bathing of persons with mental or physical disabilities requires considerable knowledge and skill. A wide variety of design features, supplies, and equipment is now available. If methods are individualized (Table 10.5) bathing can be a markedly enhanced experience for both bather and caregiver.

REFERENCES

Brawley, E. C. (1997). *Designing for Alzheimer's disease: Strategies for creating better care environments* (pp. 45, 97, 196–202). New York: John Wiley & Sons, Inc.

Day, K., Carreon, D., & Stump, C. (2000). The therapeutic design of environments for people with dementia: A review of the empirical research. *The Gerontologist, 40*(4), 397–416.

Mann, W. C., Hurren, D., Tomita, M., & Charvat, B. (1996). Use of assistive devices for bathing by elderly who are not institutionalized. *The Occupational Therapy Journal of Research, 16*(4), 261–284.

Sloane, P. D., Honn, V. J., Dwyer, S. A. R., Wieselquist, J., Cain, C., & Myers, S. (1995, July/August). Bathing the Alzheimer's patient in long-term care: Results and recommendations from three studies. *The American Journal of Alzheimer's Disease,* 3–11.

Sloane, P. D., Rader, J., Barrick, A., Hoeffer, B., Dwyer, S., McKenzie, D., Lavelle, M., Buckwalter, K., Arrington, L., & Pruitt, T. (1995). Bathing persons with dementia. *The Gerontologist, 33*(5), 672–678.

Teresi, J. A., Holmes, D., & Ory, M. G. (2000). Commentary: The therapeutic design of environments for people with dementia: Further reflections and recent findings from the National Institute on Aging collaborative studies of dementia special care units. *The Gerontologist, 40*(4), 417–421.

Warner, M. L. (2000). *The complete guide to Alzheimer's proofing your home* (pp. 24, 165–171, 321–331, 387–399). Indiana: Purdue University Press.

APPENDIX

Resources

Alzheimer's Association
919 North Michigan Ave, Suite 1100
Chicago, IL 60611-1676
(312) 335-8700
(800) 272-3900
FAX (312) 335-1110
www.alz.org

Arjo, Inc.
50 North Gary Ave.
Roselle, IL 60172
(800) 323-1245
FAX 1-888-594-2756
www.arjousa.com

Bed-Side, Inc.
PO Box 580422
2123 9th St., Suite 201
Tuslaloosa, AL 35403
(281) 333-4424
(888) 233-4424
FAX (281) 333-4005
www.bed-side.com

Briggs Corporation
PO Box 1698
Des Moines, IA 50306-9874
(800) 247-2343
FAX 1-800-222-1996
www.BriggsCorp.com

CareScout
36 Washington St. Suite 250
Wellesley Hills, MA 02481
1-781-431-7033
FAX 1-781-431-7034
www.carescout.com

Comfort Bath, Sage Products Inc.
815 Tek Dr.
PO Box 9693
Crystal Lake, IL 60014-9693
(877) 926-6367
www.comfortbath.com

ConvaQuip, Bariatric Equipment
PO Box 3417
Abilene, TX 79604
(800) 637-8436
FAX (915) 677-7217
www.convaquip.com

Disability Products Inc.
(877) 703-7499
www.adv-safety.com
info@disability-products.com

Diversified Fiberglass Fabrications, Inc.
The Ultimate in Bathing Features
1405 Hwy. 150 West
Cherryville, NC 28021
(704) 435-9586
FAX (704) 435-9596
www.dffinc.com
dffinc@vnet.net

Elite Home Medical Supplies
706 W. Lumsden Rd.
Brandon, FL 33510
(800) 229-9600
www.elitemedical.com

Incline Technologies, INC.
PO Box 4848
Incline Village, NV 89450
(702) 832-2500
(800) 538-0205
FAX (702) 832-2525
www.inclinetechnologies.com

Invacare Corporation
One Invacare Way
Elyria, OH 44036-2125
(800) 333-6900
www.invacare.com

Luxury Bath Systems, Inc.
232 James St.
Bensenville, IL 60106
(800) 354-2284
www.luxurybath.com

National Bathing Products
5 Greenwood Ave.
Romeoville, IL 60446
(815) 886-5900
www.nationalbath.com

Silcraft Corporation
528 Hughes Dr.
Traverse City, MI 49686
(800) 678-7100
www.silcraft.com

Venco
Unit # 124 - North 3808 Sullivan Rd
Spokane, WA 99216
(509) 927-2280
FAX (509) 927-4957
www.vencoproducts.com

Part III

Supporting Caregiving Activities

CHAPTER 11

Organizing Care Within the Institution or Home

Joanne Rader, Darlene McKenzie,
Beverly Hoeffer, and Ann Louise Barrick

If you are a family caregiver, you most likely have a great deal to say about how care is provided in your home. If you are a caregiver in a long-term care facility, your voice may be one of many. Organizational values will influence whose voice is heard when change is an issue. How do you become a champion of change?

ORGANIZATIONAL VALUES: WHAT NEEDS TO BE IN PLACE

Team Approach to Caregiving

Decision-Making Role of the Person

Nowhere in admission papers does it say that when you walk through the doors and become a resident of a care facility that you give up the right to refuse care or to maintain your independence. Yet, that is the experience of many persons with and without dementia, related to bathing. In the philosophy and values represented in this book, the person receiving care retains those rights, and caregivers are charged with figuring out how to present and provide care that individuals will agree to and if possible enjoy. The goals are to keep decision making very close to the resident and to help that person maintain the highest possible level of independence and function. These goals create a tightrope on which caregivers must walk when working with a person with cognitive loss. They must respect the autonomy and independence of the residents, yet make sure they receive the care they need and assistance with decisions.

Decision-Making Role of the Direct Caregiver

Currently the direct care provider (the person doing the day-to-day care activities) has many names: certified nursing assistant (CNA), resident assistant, universal worker, service partner, and personal care assistant, to name a few. The amount of training these workers are required to have varies from setting to setting and state to state. Some must take a month-long class and others are trained on the job.

This book describes a philosophy that supports direct caregivers having authority, autonomy, and flexibility to adapt when and how people are bathed. For this to work and be safe, the philosophy also assumes that direct caregivers will be accountable and responsible. For example, if a resident refuses a bath or shower, our approach expects that the caregiver will try a variety of approaches to get the person to agree (getting him or her to "yes"). If the person still refuses, then the caregiver needs to determine what must be cleaned for compelling health reasons and have the skills to identify and carry out the most pleasant, least invasive way to do it. If the decision is to postpone the bath, then an alternative plan needs to be developed. The situation of a "bath refusal" is not as difficult to manage when caregivers are consistently assigned to a group of people. But in any situation, it is not enough for the caregiver to simply say, "I asked her and she said 'no.' It's her choice. There is nothing I can do."

Caregivers have frequently reported to the authors (Rader and Barrick) that if they try to adapt, postpone, or shorten bathing, they feel judged by their peers and supervisors. In the current culture their attempts to individualize the bath are sometimes seen as an attempt to "get out of work." This attitude needs to change.

If the job is viewed strictly as a number of tasks to be completed on a group of bodies (washing, dressing, feeding, changing) day after day, there is little reward and caregiving will be seen as an unattractive field of work. If instead, the job is viewed and supported as an opportunity to enter into meaningful and caring relationships with people in need of assistance, it provides a way to be of service to others, and can be quite attractive. To recruit and retain good caregivers, the organizational system should be set up to support relationship and caring. If an organizational system is not designed with these goals in mind, a lot of money and effort will be spent on recruiting, training, orienting, and retraining people entering and exiting through a revolving door.

The person providing the hands-on care is at the center of good care along with the person receiving care (Figure 11.1), but both are often left out of care-planning. The direct caregiver has unique knowledge, access and responsibility for care. However, this knowledge may be ignored or not sought in the care-planning process. For example, direct caregivers are typically excluded from attending care-planning conferences. This is because they are seen as "too busy." Plus, unless their input is sought and used, caregivers may feel attendance is a waste of their time. Often, the staff members attending the conference don't have the same daily, direct access to the residents. We have made progress through the Omnibus Budget Reconciliation Act of 1987 in including families and residents in care planning. We need to do the same for direct caregivers.

Supportive Role of the Supervisor

In light of the growing workforce shortage, changing roles, and changing health care systems, it is time to rethink how direct caregivers are supervised. Often, in care facilities, the person who is overseeing direct caregivers is a nurse. In nursing homes a nurse is available in the building around the clock. In assisted living, adult foster care, or residential care, the nurse serves in a more consultative role and may not always be present in the building.

Much of the nurse's time currently is tied up doing paperwork and very little is spent at the bedside. The old relationship model between the nurse and the direct care provider is reflected in the commonly used title "nursing assistant," which implies that they are there to help the nurse complete her job, which has been defined as providing and overseeing the care of a group of people. The role and responsibilities in this dynamic are changing with the licensed nurse moving further from the bedside. Much more of the decision making and problem solving is falling to direct care workers because they are at the bedside.

Despite this shift, many nurses are still supervising in the old model where they "know best." Thus there can be a discrepancy between the degree of support nurses feel they provide to direct caregivers and the amount of support caregivers feel they receive. CNAs sometimes view nurses as being critical and lacking understanding about residents' needs and wishes. For example, one CNA reported to the nurse that she had tried various approaches with a person to get her to agree to a shower. From her knowledge of the person, she knew any shower today would result in a battle. She shared this information with the nurse who told her to shower her anyway. The person was showered and the situation became a battle, ending with both CNA and resident exhausted and distressed. On seeing them exit the shower the nurse said to the resident, "There, don't you feel better now that you are clean?"

We propose a supervising model (Figure 11.1) that more closely reflects the new relationship between the nurse and direct caregiver. Here, in the center of the circle, is the person being cared for. Surrounding the person receiving care are the direct caregivers. Those individuals on the outside of the circle, which includes nurses, are in service to those in the middle. That is, nurses figure out how they can best assist the direct caregiver in providing good care. Thus, they support rather than simply direct.

This "new" model can work. One facility in Oregon had a nurse manager who operated out of this model and demonstrated the benefits. She respected the knowledge and skills of the CNAs; she routinely provided resources such as education, modeling, and verbal support. She understood the need for the CNAs to be decision makers, having flexibility and choice about how care was delivered. She also held them accountable for providing good care. She stood up for them with administration to assure they had what they needed to provide good care. For example, initially there was resistance for purchasing a no-rinse soap product and another product was ordered. The CNAs tried it, but felt it was inferior to the first product. The nurse worked with administration until the no-rinse product the CNAs initially recom-

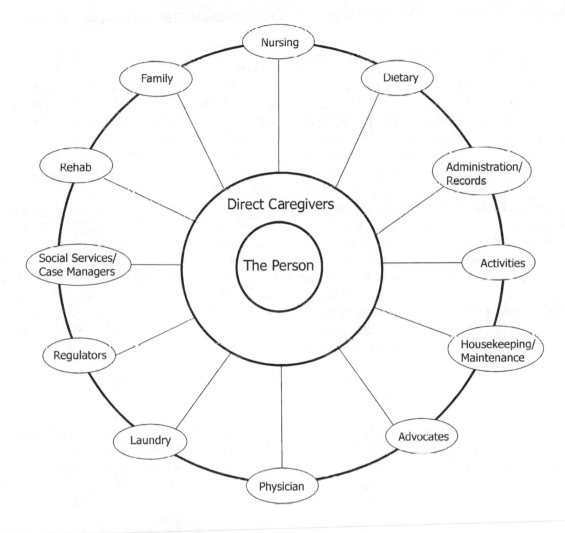

FIGURE 11.1   At the center of good care.

Note. From "At the Hub of Good Care," 1999, *Nursing Assistant Monthly, 5*(3), p. 1. Adapted and reprinted with permission from Frontline Publishing, P.O. Box 441002, Somerville, MA 02144. For more information, call (800) 348-0605.

mended was ordered. That soap is now a standard product in the facility.

In addition, with this same nurse's support and knowledge, a very skilled CNA began teaching her colleagues what she knew about bathing. She worked with other staff to individualize bathing for all residents on the dementia unit, greatly reducing the agitation and distress experienced during bathing. Now, this nursing assistant is considered the "bathing expert" in the facility. With the supervising nurse's encouragement, she consults with other units in the facility. In addition, she now copresents at conferences with the author (Rader) on bathing without a battle.

Not all direct care workers are motivated and skilled at working with people with dementia. Some need help dealing with care refusals or identifying and implementing alternate plans for bathing. Part of the supervisor's job is to educate, model and support positive staff behaviors. In addition, it is also necessary to identify where improvement is needed and set up a plan of correction.

Not everyone is suited for caregiving work. Those who are not, whether they are nurses, direct care workers or others, should be encouraged to move on. This is a hard thing to do when staffing shortages are so acute, but people who don't have a knack for the work often just create more work for others and discomfort for the people in their care.

Continuity in Bathing Care

Consistent Assignments vs. Rotation

Staffing patterns are crucial in determining the quality of the bathing experience. We have discussed the importance of having the same person doing the bathing. This can be accomplished in several ways. Many facilities have switched to what is called consistent or permanent assignments for staff. This means that a direct caregiver on each shift is assigned to care for the same group of people over time. On his/her days off, a consistent associate caregiver will fill in. The idea is to have as few people as possible providing care to each person. Other caregivers in the facility or the unit will also need to know about the individual so they can fill in when needed and the primary caregiver can provide information that can be passed on by word of mouth and also in the care plan. Direct caregivers that have worked under this system generally come to prefer it. The benefits they identify are:

- Caregivers get to know the residents and their preferred routines better.
- Caregivers experience closer, more meaningful relationships with the recipients of their care, resulting in more overall job satisfaction.
- Families know whom to ask for information.
- Good caregivers or poor caregivers becomes readily apparent.
- Fewer items such as clothing, grooming articles, or assistive devices get lost.

Some problems can occur with a system of consistent or permanent assignments. Staff members may become very attached to certain individuals. When these individuals become ill and die, staff members may feel like they have lost a family member. Therefore, these circumstances need to be anticipated and addressed. For example, arrangements may need to be made so staff can attend funerals. Some kind of ceremony or way of honoring deaths can be established within the facility. Staff need to know it is all right to cry and grieve these deaths. Sometimes a staff member can become too possessive of a person with dementia. Then, the role of the supervisor is to help them sort out what is best for the person. From the resident's perspective, the departure of a favorite staff member can be a painful and difficult situation. Again, this situation needs to

be anticipated. These problems grow out of caring. Wouldn't you rather be bathed by someone who cares rather than someone who is just performing a task on a body?

Avoid having caregivers rotate between groups of people on a weekly or monthly basis. Although this method of staffing is still used in many places, it does not create consistency and is becoming outdated. Sometimes caregivers initially say they prefer this system so they don't get "burned out" on someone. When a change towards more consistency in assignments is suggested, comments such as "I couldn't stand to take care of some of them for more than a week" are sometimes heard. Facilities that have made the switch to permanent or consistent assignments find that different caregivers prefer different types of people. If caregivers are allowed choice in assignments, it usually works out well. If they become frustrated with caring for someone after a time, ways can be established for them to shift to another assignment.

Focused Assignment on Bathing

Another method used to create continuity in bathing is to **have a caregiver whose sole task is to bathe people.** They are usually called "bath aides." Because they do not have other care tasks to do, they often have a lot of flexibility in terms of time of day (within their assigned shift) or day of the week that bathing can be done. In addition, many bath aides take a great deal of pride in creating a pleasant experience for the person and are very skilled at their craft. Unless these individuals get pulled from their bathing duties because of staff call-ins or shortages, this method usually provides consistency.

One disadvantage of using bath aides is that they bathe throughout the shift. Thus, the time of day the person is being bathed may seem a bit odd, such as right before lunch after he/she is already dressed for the day. Another disadvantage is that if the bath aide is assigned to work on the floor instead of bathing, the task of bathing then falls to another aide. The newly assigned aide may not be familiar with the person's desired routine, particular needs and wishes. Additionally, the newly assigned aide may not possess the same level of bathing skills as the original bath aide. Also, when care is being done by a variety of persons who are each assigned to do particular tasks, it is sometimes more difficult to focus on the person before the task and coordinate all required care activities.

There are many ways that staff can be assigned to bathe residents. The goal should be to have consistent and caring people with the ability to adjust the time of day, day of the week, and method to meet the person's wishes and changing needs.

Commitment to Individualized Bathing Care

Methods of Bathing

The caregiver needs to be able to adjust **how** a person is bathed. This requires moment-by-moment decisions about the best ways to get a person clean. All the variations described in previous chapters should be considered potential ways for bathing. These include such options as: in-bed and in-room bathing, bathing in the shower using a no-rinse soap, and dividing up the bathing into smaller tasks. In addition, physical and occupational therapists should be available to help in figuring out how to adapt the method of bathing and the environment to be more supportive.

Flexibility in Bathing

Hands-on caregivers' time is the most precious commodity in the care environment. Facilities might find it useful to question old patterns and rituals that may not be the best use of time. The most common way that care facilities assign a bath or shower is by establishing a routine number of times a week it is to be done, and assigning residents to particular days of the week and time of day (shift). The most common routine appears to be twice-weekly baths or showers. This number is not based on any hard evidence, but is generally accepted practice. This "sacred cow" needs to be reevaluated. Frequency of baths should be individualized. Persons who are incontinent, perspire heavily, or spill food require frequent freshening up for good health and skin care. However, washing the entire body and hair twice a week may be unnecessary. In several facilities in North Carolina and Oregon, many people were bathed for three months using a no-rinse soap solution and were not rinsed or washed with running water. No untoward clinical effects from either reducing the number of baths or eliminating the running water were observed.

This raises an interesting question: **Are we using direct-caregivers' precious time to do a procedure that many residents do not enjoy, more often than is necessary or desired, simply because it is "the way we have always done it?"** Doesn't it make more sense to look at an individual's preferences and needs to determine how and when bathing will occur? Some people may desire and need less frequent bathing while others prefer to bathe daily. Meeting these wishes becomes more plausible with flexibility. Supervisors of direct caregivers must rethink their roles and allow responsible caregivers the autonomy and flexibility to redefine the cleansing experience.

Case Study

Here is a case study that illustrates a facility that has implemented the change necessary to individualize bathing:

> Helen is consistently assigned to Mrs. Jonson, who is usually bathed on Saturday. However, this Saturday Helen is sick and Mrs. Jonson wishes to wait until Helen returns to get her shower. This wish is honored. The caregiver filling in invites another resident to shower instead, to lighten the load for Helen when she returns. Helen will do her best to get Mrs. Jonson showered the day she returns, but if that is not possible she will negotiate with her, being sure that necessary parts are washed to prevent problems.

Case Discussion

In this facility individualized bathing and teamwork are valued. Mrs. Johnson's wishes are more important than getting a bath on a designated day. Caregivers work together, adjusting their schedules, helping each other. Helen recognizes that Mrs. Jonson likes the routine that they have worked out in the shower where she is bathed with a no-rinse soap and is not sprayed with the hose. She also knows that she has the support of her supervisor who will be more concerned about honoring Mrs. Jonson's wishes than whether or not she is bathed on a particular day. Because of the relationship they have built, Helen knows that Mrs. Jonson trusts she will do all she can to shower her when she returns and make it a pleasant experience.

HOW TO MOVE A FACILITY FORWARD

So where do you begin if you want to implement change? Someone needs to champion the process of individualizing bathing. It is best if this person is at least in a supervisory position. If you are a direct caregiver, you could share your thoughts and this book with your supervisor or another person in authority who can help implement the change process. Certainly there is much you can do as an individual during each bath, but if you want more far-reaching effects, you will need to partner with others. If you are a supervisor or director of nursing, approach administration to ensure that you have support to begin a process of trying new ideas. Administration may need to approve costs related to supplies and training. In addition, you will want to involve the direct caregivers in the planning process. The following ideas support one format, but there are many different ways to implement change. Crafting a formula that fits you, your role, and your facility is of utmost importance. Here are the suggested steps:

- **Focus on exploring and trying different methods of bathing as a good first step.**
  Begin by trying some of the techniques mentioned in this book, such as covering during the shower, washing the hair last, and using the towel bath so you are familiar with them. Using different methods is a fairly concrete and easy way to begin.

- **Start on one unit to work through details and solutions.**
  - Pick the unit that you feel would be the most supportive, looking at the quality of the teamwork.
  - Start by having a discussion with the direct caregivers and ask them to identify people who dislike being bathed and/or who display resistive behaviors so the range of problems is known.
  - Do an inservice (see suggested outline in chapter 12) to familiarize staff with options.
  - Pick one resident (it is best not to start with the worst case, but the simplest).
  - Ask for staff volunteers to try new options. It is helpful to have two people involved so they can problem solve together.
  - If you are championing the change, you might also want to be present to provide support or feedback. Keep in mind that too many people in the room may be overwhelming and frightening to the resident.

- You may want one caregiver to videotape the bath or shower. Such tapes are very useful in identifying triggers for distress and new approaches to try. They can also be used to demonstrate the effectiveness of individualized bathing approaches. Videotaping requires permission of all involved as well as care to protect the confidentiality and privacy of the persons being videotaped. Since these tapes contain very sensitive material, only caregivers involved, other direct caregivers on the unit, and the supervisor would normally view the tape. In some situations, however, you may want to obtain the explicit permission to show the tape to others in the facility for educational purposes. These tapes should be erased after viewing.
- Continue the trial and error process until your goals are achieved. Chapter 4 gives some tools for identifying and measuring goals.
- Repeat this process with another resident.
- Set up a Quality Improvement Program (see Appendix A for suggestions).

- **Address the larger, system issues that affect bathing.**
  At this point, you may be encountering questions and obstacles related to frequency of bathing, staffing patterns, and the role of the caregiver and supervisor. Clearly, changing the way we think about and practice bathing influences many elements of the care system. It is important to address the big-picture issues as they emerge.

  - Set up a committee or group to help identify problems and solutions.
  - Estimate a budget for any equipment needs (towels, no-rinse soap).
  - Look at staffing patterns to see if they support or hinder change.
  - "Protect" direct caregivers' workload to ensure time for flexibility.
  - Establish systematic review and evaluation of individualized bathing approaches. For example, the question of a person's bathing comfort and distress could be addressed at each quarterly care-planning conference.
  - Reward direct caregivers for their role in improving care. This can take many forms in-

cluding having them take an active role in inservice and training. It should also be a part of their performance evaluation. Give out an award to the person who discovered the best way to bathe a complex resident.

- Develop methods for including the philosophy and specifics about individualized bathing into orientation for staff, particularly direct caregivers and nurses. If you have a CNA training program, be sure that what is taught is consistent with what you want to see in practice.
- Incorporate the individualized bathing philosophy into orientation and facility introduction information given to families and residents.
- Include accomplishments and needs routinely in reports to administration.
- Regularly post any quality assurance data you have (protecting confidentiality) so that caregivers and others can monitor progress.

Bathing can serve as a catalyst for improving care in general. Facilities are increasingly being put in the position of having to rethink the basic organization of care in order to meet the changing needs and demands of the consumers, so reevaluating your methods and philosophy of bathing can assist with this.

- **Be proactive with regulators (surveyors, etc.) and advocates.**

  - Let them know the positive things you are doing to improve practice.
  - Ask them to share any questions or concerns.
  - Invite them to visit and observe.

- **Have your new "experts" on the unit do an inservice for the facility and families to share successes and solutions.**

  - Use any data you have collected to demonstrate your progress.
  - Use direct caregivers as coinstructors and have them demonstrate new techniques that they have found useful.
  - Set up ways for those who have been successful to consult with other units who are implementing change.

- Encourage the other units to follow a similar process to create change on the unit.

BATHING AT HOME

The organizational issues for families caring for persons with dementia at home are different than those for caregivers in facilities. Usually, just one caregiver is caring for the person at home, thus providing continuity in an already existing relationship. However, being a solitary caregiver can be tiring and overwhelming, causing anger and frustration as a result of the stress experienced. The bathing experience may then feel like a battle, particularly if the person resists your efforts to help. Taking care of yourself is as important as taking care of your family member with dementia as explained in chapter 13.

Sometimes family members or friends wanting to be helpful may give advice or criticism without recognizing the complexity of the situation. Instead, what you need from members of your family and friendship network is someone you can talk with about your situation, concrete help with specific tasks and activities, and occasional respite from caregiving. For example, a friend or other family member could do the shopping, pick up medications, or take over some household chores or assistance with personal care activities such as bathing. Your ability to reach out and ask for assistance is very important to your health. If your health fails or you become overwhelmed, your ability to provide care at home to your family member will be compromised.

Thinking Creatively About Bathing

Family members also need to examine their own myths about keeping people clean. Again, beliefs that people must have a shower or tub bath to get clean limit options and create unnecessarily upsetting situations for both of you. For many reasons, bathing can be overwhelming for the person. Many of the ideas discussed in chapters 2, 3, and 4 are very adaptable to the home setting. Here are some additional ideas to think about.

Shared Bathing

Sometimes spouses or partners find it helpful and easy to join the person in the shower and bathe together. If this is an acceptable option for you, it can provide a time of caring and intimacy that both of you will find pleasurable.

Adult Children as Caregivers

When an adult child takes on the role of bathing a parent, it can be emotionally difficult, particularly if the caregiver is the opposite sex of the person being bathed. At first the change of roles may feel awkward and uncomfortable. Using humor can often make the situation easier for all.

Sometimes, if the person with dementia doesn't recognize the adult child or thinks he/she is the spouse, the person may make sexual comments or advances that feel inappropriate or distressing. Some family members have chosen to stop assisting with bathing because of their distress related to such behaviors. However, these actions need to be looked at in the context of the illness that is causing the disorientation and disinhibition. Persons with dementia may say and do things that are completely out of context for them because their "censor functions" no longer work. Clarifying to the person who you are and setting limits can be helpful in some cases. For example, you could say "Dad, I'm your daughter. Please stop."

Using Outside Resources to Help

Hiring someone to come into the home to provide assistance with bathing, perhaps along with providing respite to you as the caregiver, can be very beneficial to both. If you feel the person may be resistant to having someone else help with personal care, start out with the hired caregiver coming in and getting to know the person first. Look for someone with experience in working with persons who have dementia. You are looking for a caregiver who can help get the person to "yes" and adapt bathing to the needs of the person. For example, some hired in-home caregivers report that they have bathed people quite well while they were sitting in a recliner.

The bathrooms in the home may be small and may or may not be adapted to meet changing physical and emotional needs. Chapter 9 has good information about how to adapt the bathroom to make it a friendlier, safer place.

Conclusion

Changing the way care is thought about and delivered can be a challenge especially in organizational settings. But even at home most of us are used to providing care in certain ways, and changing can be hard to do. This chapter discusses some of the important issues to consider and provides a framework for creating change. Direct caregivers such as nursing assistants are limited in their ability to implement change without supervisory and administrative support, yet they and the person with dementia have to carry the burden if organizational support for change is lacking. One author (Rader) was doing an inservice at a facility that was attended by nursing assistants only, no nurses or managers. When finished, one CNA spoke up and said, "What good does it do for us to hear this if the nurses aren't here?" She was right. She knew that without the buy-in of administration and supervisors, no significant change would be possible or sustainable. Equally true, if you are the supervising nurse, you must have the support of the direct caregivers. As a change agent, you need to be aware of the need for partners to assist you in the process.

Individualizing the bathing experience for persons with dementia can serve as a model for creating system change, resulting in greater job satisfaction for staff. Providing individualized care fosters trust, a very real commodity in the caregiving relationship. When caregivers are put in the position of having to bathe someone against his/her will, it destroys trust that takes time and energy to develop. They may "harden their hearts" and turn bathing into merely a task to be done because it is too painful to continually do something that they know is perceived as an assault by the person being cared for. This can lead to caregiver frustration, burnout, and turnover. For this reason and others discussed in this book, unless there is a compelling health reason, people should not be bathed against their will. To do so borders on abuse. Although changing bathing practices may not be easy, the benefits for the relationship are worth it!

CHAPTER 12

Training Staff in Ways to Keep People Clean

Joyce H. Rasin, Ann Louise Barrick,
and Joanne Rader

Two of the fundamental values in the bathing approach discussed in previous chapters are individualization of the bathing process and the importance of the relationship between the care provider and the care receiver. These values are also important in the approach to training care providers. In the individualization of bathing, the care provider recognizes that the care recipient has preferred ways of getting clean. Instructors in a training situation must also be aware that participants have preferred ways of learning. Likewise, the interaction between instructor and participant is just as important as the care provider-care receiver interaction. The effective instructor is sensitive and responds to the needs of the participant. Further responses are influenced by feedback received from the participant. This chapter will discuss how to create a supportive learning environment, suggest teaching strategies that are appropriate for different learning styles, and describe the necessary components of clinical learning.

CREATING A SUPPORTIVE LEARNING ENVIRONMENT

The instructor must take the lead in setting the tone for the class in order to maximize participants' motivation to learn. A positive learning environment is emotionally and physically comfortable and communicates respect for participants.

Creating Comfort

Icebreakers and warm-up exercises are useful for creating a comfortable learning environment. Even when participants know each other, warm-up activities can encourage involvement and interaction. They help participants get to know each other and the instructor, and they establish the emotional climate for the class. One good warm-up exercise is to ask participants to name one thing they would like to learn during the class. The instructor can review these expectations with the group and explain how their learning goals fit into the planned material. Knowing the concerns of the group can also help the instructor adapt the information to the needs of the group as much as possible. If participants have learning goals that will not be addressed in the class, these goals might be good suggestions for developing future classes.

Communicating Respect

It is also important for the instructor to communicate respect for participants at all times. A basic rule of thumb to follow is that there is never a dumb question or response. Accept and value all responses that are made in the spirit of learning. The response may contain incorrect information, but the instructor can acknowledge the participation and clarify the information. Active listening is the most important communication skill for demonstrating respect, acceptance, and interest. It is also important to be aware of nonverbal behavior that may communicate a lack of attention, such as glancing away, interrupting a participant, and lack of eye contact. Keep in mind, however, that participants' cultural background must be taken into account when determining what nonverbal behavior communicates interest or disinterest.

Motivating the Adult Learner

Individuals need to be motivated if learning is to occur. This poses a dilemma. Many inservice classes are mandatory. Although people can be forced to attend, they may not be motivated to learn. The instructor has to work harder initially to engage the reluctant participant with low motivation. Consider the following factors when attempting to enhance participants' motivation.

Usefulness of Information

The participant must see a use for the material presented. Adults need to know why they should learn new information. If the usefulness is not apparent interest may be low. Capture the attention of the participants in the beginning of the session by describing how the topic relates to the skills needed for their work. Many care providers find that bathing individuals with dementia is difficult and problematic, so one effective strategy would be to ask the participants if they experience any problems when bathing residents.

Elicit discussion of care providers' prior experiences and link something from their experience to some new piece of information. Although this is most desirable it may not always be possible. Some old experiences should not be reinforced. Your staff may have been involved in activities in previous employment that reflect old practice standards or just misinformation. Resistance to accepting new information can be due to a negative evaluation of its usefulness based on prior experiences. Knowing about divergent viewpoints provides the trainer with an excellent opportunity to engage the learner in some problem solving and show how it can be currently applied.

Caregiver Wisdom

Most care aides were taught to start washing from the top (the hair) down. This just upsets people with dementia so I go with what is least upsetting to them, maybe their face, maybe their feet. We have to teach that it is OK to alter how you wash people to meet their needs.

Kathy House, CNA, Fairlawn Good Samaritan Health Center, Gresham, OR

Applicability

The information needs to be not only useful but also readily applicable to specific work situations. Motivation to learn increases when adult participants have a problem to solve. They want to know how information can be used with specific real-life problems and prefer that which is concrete and practical. Providing active learning exercises such as role-plays (see next section) clearly demonstrate the applicability of the material and increases learner participation. Furthermore, active learning exercises are most appropriate for teaching a process such as bathing.

Incentives

Incentives can be both psychological and tangible. Emphasize that learning about individualized bathing will make the experience more pleasurable for both the care provider and the care receiver. Tangible incentives such as refreshments and door prizes also increase interest. The incentives don't have to be costly. Most participants appreciate simply having a beverage or small door prize. Multicolored ink pens, pocket tablets, and hand lotion are useful and inexpensive, and can be tied to some aspect of the training. Make the process of distributing the prizes fun, so participants' associate a pleasurable experience with learning.

Positive Feelings

Clearly communicating the usefulness of the material, providing an opportunity to apply the material successfully, and providing incentives for learning will help participants feel positive about their experience. Positive feelings are very powerful motivators for learning and contribute to participant's feelings of self-confidence and competence.

COMPONENTS OF CLINICAL TEACHING

Acquiring new skills can be broken into two components—obtaining information about the skill and supervised practice to become competent in the skill. Although both components are needed for proficiency, continuing education programs tend to emphasize only the knowledge component. This section focuses on methods for providing information as well as the role of supervised practice.

Providing Information

Individuals acquire new information and skills in different ways. As an instructor, you will have participants who have different learning needs. One teaching method will not be suitable for all participants. Just as the care provider must have an assortment of approaches to use when working with a care receiver, the instructor should know multiple techniques for teaching and the range of possible learning needs in order to individualize teaching. In this section, specific teaching strategies are described. In the table that follows, guidelines are provided for selecting strategies that match different learning styles.

Teaching Strategies

- Lecture—This method is most frequently used in a classroom setting. It allows the instructor to provide a lot of information at one time to a large number of people. One negative aspect of lecture is that participant participation is limited, which prevents participants from learning to problem solve. Also, remembering lecture information is generally difficult unless participants are taking notes.
- Visual Aids—When you don't have the real thing, because of cost or unavailability, drawings, photographs, overheads, or models can be substituted. These can be very effective when accompanied by clear explanations. Combining visual aids with lecture (i.e., illustrated lecture) is an effective way to provide lots of information in an organized manner while maintaining participants' attention and enhancing their ability to learn the material.
- Audiovisual Aids—Materials such as videotapes or slides are a good supplement to other methods such as lecture or discussion. When a demonstration or role-play is not feasible, videotape or slides provide a good substitute. Be sure to take time to plan how the audiovisuals will be used within the lecture, especially when using them for the first time. Rehearse with the equipment and your notes so that you can do both smoothly. Video-

tapes can be used in place of an instructor when trying to reach staff members who are not available when the class is taught (e.g., due to sickness, day off, another shift). However, if the staff has no opportunity to have questions answered and concerns clarified, learning and proper implementation can be compromised. "Solving Bathing Problems in Persons with Alzheimer's Disease" is a videotape that can augment the teaching of the individualized bathing approach (see resources in chapter appendix).

- Discussion—Either lecture or videotapes may be used to elicit questions that lead to discussion. Discussion gives participants an opportunity to exchange ideas. The interchange of ideas among participants provides substantial benefits to individual participants, including learning from the experiences of others and sharing different perspectives on the application of materials.
- Demonstration—In a demonstration, you show and explain the steps of a task to the learner (e.g., towel bath or transferring) or show how to use a piece of equipment (e.g., bath chair). Because the learner uses both vision and hearing, memory and understanding are enhanced. The following steps are suggested for preparing a demonstration:

  - Obtain all of the items that you will use, and make sure any equipment you may use is working properly before the demonstration.
  - Make sure everyone can see and hear you clearly from any location in the room.
  - Before you start the demonstration, summarize what you will be doing.
  - List each step in sequence.
  - Talk through each step.
  - If possible, allow each participant to perform the task (i.e., return demonstration).

- Role-plays—Role-plays will facilitate participants' learning of the individualized bathing approach. Individualization means the caregiver has to be comfortable trying different approaches. Role-playing gives the learner a chance to think on the spot and practice different approaches in a safe environment. The trainer assists the learner in developing problem solving skills. The following steps are suggested for developing a role-play:

- Write a description of a bathing scenario. This could be a combination of some past experiences. Describe the characteristics of the care provider and the care receiver.
- Brief each participant on his or her role individually.
- Allow the scene to evolve for 5–10 minutes. The length of time will vary with the participants.
- If the participants are shy or get stuck, ask the rest of the class to provide suggestions.

- Case Study—Provide a written description of a situation that the caregivers might actually experience. This should be a realistic example, one in which the learner could imagine him or herself. The instructor can then involve all participants in problem solving and identifying possible solutions.

Matching Teaching Strategies to Learning Styles of Participants

The instructor needs to decide which strategy is appropriate for the type of material that is being presented and the learning needs of the participants. The most effective approach for trying to use teaching strategies that match the learning style of all participants in the class is to employ a variety of approaches. The diversity of techniques will improve teaching the individualized bathing approach since they will capture the interest of participants in different ways and reinforce material that is important to learn. Suggested teaching styles for specific learning styles are in Table 12.1. A list of in-service classes for teaching individualized bathing and a sample training module that illustrates the use of a variety of teaching strategies is in the chaper appendix.

Supervised Practice

If skills that were learned in the classroom are not practiced, they will quickly be forgotten. A care provider might be reluctant to perform a new skill independently until he/she can develop both competence and confidence. Supervised practice fosters accurate mastery of skills because the care provider has the opportunity to perform the task or skill under the watchful eye of an experienced provider. Peers working as mentors/

TABLE 12.1 Suggested Teaching Strategies

Learning Style	Teaching Strategies
VERBAL PARTICIPANTS need spoken or written presentations.	Lecture, handout, case study.
VISUAL PARTICIPANTS need visual presentations of material rather that verbal descriptions.	Demonstrations, illustrations, handouts, visual aids, videotape. Pictures and illustrations help participants to learn and to recall the information. In teaching about the bathing process, the visual learner would appreciate a handout with the procedure described, step-by-step, with pictures. The pictures could be very simple stick figures.
SEQUENTIAL LEARNERS are participants who prefer learning material by breaking it down into small steps.	Visual aids that include step-by-step instructions such as handouts, overheads, or demonstrations. The knowledge of the specific methods to get people clean is important for mastery of the bathing approach, and this type of material is quite conducive to a sequential presentation.
TOP-DOWN OR CONTEXTUAL PARTICIPANTS need to see the big picture before mastering the details. They want to know how the new information fits into their world.	Provide a written outline of the material to be discussed at the beginning of the workshop. Incorporate participants' personal experiences (e.g., show that their desires/needs during bathing don't differ from the person with dementia; ask the participants what makes bathing enjoyable for them; connect their experiences to the experience of persons with dementia). Provide an overall context for the material (e.g., emphasize that individualized bathing is not only a procedure to get someone clean, but is one part of an overall approach to interacting with persons who have dementia).
EXPERIENTIAL PARTICIPANTS like to be actively engaged with new information. They remember better if they can be physically involved.	Demonstrations, role-play. Have them physically interact by handling the bathing supplies and actually practicing the bath. If possible, videotape them in role-play or bathing situation, and review the tape together.

coaches can perform this role. The purpose of the clinical mentor or coach is to help the mentee to apply the new skill in the clinical setting. The mentor should initially model the appropriate behaviors and then provide guidance as the mentee tries out the new skill. The ideal mentor/coach is an expert in both clinical practice and teaching clinical skills. Specifically, the mentor/coach should be comfortable and competent with using an individualized bathing approach and should be able to teach these skills to an adult learner. The training skills include learning about teaching adult participants and stimulating motivation and confidence. Acquiring the necessary training skills requires that new mentors/coaches also receive mentoring initially.

Caregiver Wisdom

As a designated mentor, I talk with the new aide before we go in. I explain a little about who the person is, what he/she likes and doesn't like and the method of bathing that works best and why. Then I go in and demonstrate how to do it. After, I check to see if the aide has any questions. The next time, I help them set up and let them begin, and then I see how they are doing. If they need assistance, I role model how to resolve the situation. If they seem comfortable, I step back. I make sure I give them feedback about how well they are doing.

Beth Parker, CNA, Marian Estates, Sublimity, OR

SUMMARY

- The instructor is responsible for creating a supportive and comfortable learning environment for participants.
- To motivate adult participants, it is important to: 1) clearly communicate the usefulness of the material; 2) demonstrate the applicability of the material in everyday situations; 3) provide incentives for learning; and 4) engender participants with positive feelings such as confidence and competence.
- The instructor should be familiar with a variety of different teaching strategies that are appropriate for participants' different learning needs and styles.

- The two necessary components of clinical teaching are providing information and providing supervised practice to help participants develop skillful approaches to bathing.

APPENDIX

Training Modules

Learning programs can be developed for administrators, nurse supervisors, nursing assistants, and family caregivers. They can be developed in a modular fashion, so that some modules (or portions thereof) can serve multiple learners. Use the following list of possible learning programs and the sample training module for in-room bathing as you develop your own training program.

Outline of Training for Bathing Persons with Dementia	
Topic	Target Audience*
Providing flexible bathing opportunities for patients and staff	ADM, NRS, FAM
Promoting teamwork in the provision of personal care	ADM, NRS
Problem solving techniques that reduce agitation during bathing	NRS, DCG, FAM
Communicating with the Alzheimer's patient	ADM, NRS, DCG, FAM
Transfer techniques	NRS, DCG, FAM
Tips on successful in-room bathing	NRS, DCG, FAM
Tips on successful showering	NRS, DCG, FAM
Tips on successful tub bathing	NRS, DCG, FAM
Equipment that can assist in bathing difficult patients	ADM, NRS, FAM

*ADM = administrators; NRS = nurse supervisors; DCG = direct caregivers (e.g., nursing assistants); FAM = families

TRAINING MODULE

In-Room Bathing

Materials needed:

Blackboard, whiteboard, pad on an easel or something to write down ideas and questions

Equipment for towel bath: (enough so every pair of participants can make up a kit)
- Two or more bath blankets
- One large plastic bag containing:
  - One large, lightweight towel
  - One standard bath towel
  - Two or more washcloths
- No-rinse soap
- Plastic pitcher
- Large bath blankets

Rollaway bed

Overheads:

1. Consider a bed bath
2. Steps in the towel bath
3. Individualizing the towel bath

Handouts:

1. The Towel Bath (Table 4.4)
2. Individualizing the Towel Bath (Table 4.5)
3. Myths of bathing

Learning objectives:

1. To understand the benefits of in-room bathing.
2. To determine those persons who are appropriate for in-room bathing.
3. To acquire skill in one type of in-room bathing: the towel bath.
4. To be able to alter the towel bath in order to meet individual needs.

Outline:

1. Warm-up.
2. Discussion of some of the myths of bathing.
3. Reasons for using an in-room bathing method.
4. Demonstration of towel bath.
5. Opportunity to practice towel bath.
6. Discussion of methods of individualizing the towel bath.
7. Discussion of pros and cons of the towel bath.

Examples for instructors:

1. Warm-up: Open the session with one of these exercises to create a comfortable learning environment and encourage interaction among participants and interest in the topic.

   a. Ask participants to settle back and think about a bath or shower they particularly enjoyed. Ask them to picture being in the same bath or shower—to feel the water, smell the aromas, relive the experience in their minds. Give participants a few minutes to visualize this bath and then ask them to share with the others what made that bath enjoyable. List on the board all the factors that participants mention (e.g., warm, soothing, refreshing, relaxing, invigorating). Then ask them about bathing a person with dementia. How would they describe **a typical bath or shower** for this person (e.g., frightening, painful, cold)?

   b. Ask participants about their preferences for bathing. Use questions such as: When do you like to bath—morning, evening, both? Do you prefer a shower? A tub bath? What do you do if you don't feel like a bath or shower but know you have areas that need cleaning?

2. Discuss some of the myths of bathing (pass out handout). Specific ones to include are:

   a. It takes lots of water to rinse someone.
   b. Families will insist on a shower or bath.

Encourage discussion of alternative methods of getting clean. Ask for suggestions and write the responses on whatever you use to write down suggestions and comments. Conclude with the statement that sometimes an in-room bath in the bed is the best choice.

3. Discuss the persons who are most likely to benefit from in-room bathing and why. These include (see overhead) those who:

   - are frail and who fatigue easily;
   - are nonambulatory;
   - experience pain or transfer;
   - are fearful of lifts;
   - have acute illness;
   - are afraid of the shower spray;
   - are overstimulated in the shower;
   - are expressing the desire for it.

4. Demonstrate the towel bath (use overhead with steps). Give out handout with towel bath instructions.
5. Ask participants to pair up and prepare the towel bath. Have them mix the no-rinse soap, pour it into the bag with the towel and washcloths and feel the degree of wetness. At this point you can ask for a volunteer who is willing to put on a gown and receive a modified towel bath. The person receiving the towel bath can then give feedback to the person giving it. Ask for what feels good; what doesn't feel good. An alternative to this is to have participants practice on each other using a dry towel.
6. Case study: Use a case study to help participants understand the need to individualize the towel bath just as you would any bath (use the overhead on individualizing the towel bath to stimulate discussion).

Discussion questions:

1. What concerns do you have about using this as the primary method of bathing?
2. What would need to be in place for you to implement this in-bed bathing method?
3. How could you discuss switching from shower to in-bed bathing with the family? What points would you want to make? What possible concerns would you want to anticipate? How could you reassure them that good care will continue?

Follow-up:

The next step would be to ask for volunteers to try the towel bath with bedside consultation by the instructor. This will be an excellent opportunity to refine skills in giving the bed bath as well as assessing needs and varying the approach.

Resources

Active Learning: Some online articles and a bibliography from New York State University at Buffalo. http://ublib.buffalo.edu/libraries/projects/tlr/active.html.

Equipment: See Chapter 10.

Videotape: Solving Bathing Problems in Persons with Alzheimer's Disease and Related Dementia by Phillip Sloane, Ann Louise Barrick, and Vanessa Horn. To order contact Health Professions Press at 1-888-337-8808 or their Web site: http://www.healthpropress.com/CATALOG/videos/Bathmain.html.

BATHING WITHOUT A BATTLE: COMMON MYTHS RELATED TO BATHING

- **It takes lots of water to get people clean.**
  In health care and home settings, people have kept clean without the benefit of showers, tubs or running water. Careful washing, with attention to details, is more important than how much water you use.

- **If caregivers are delaying, deferring, shortening or adapting the bath or shower, they are trying to get out of work.**
  This may be necessary to create an individualized plan that meets the person's special needs. They are still responsible for maintaining the person's hygiene, but need freedom to adjust the method.

- **Families will insist on a shower or tub bath.**
  Families, like the rest of us, need to be educated. If they are presented with the problem (the person dislikes or fights the bath or shower) and alternative suggestions, usually they understand and are agreeable with a trial of other methods.

- **There will be more infections and skin problems.**
  Many people have not gotten into a shower or tub for years, yet they are clean and have no increased infections or skin problems.

- **People always feel better after they have a bath or shower.**
  If it is forced, people feel attacked, demoralized, fearful and it is an exhausting process.

- **You have to just go ahead because for most people who resist, there won't be a "good" time.**
  For most people with dementia, it is possible to develop a plan that keeps them clean and avoids the battle by adapting the approach, method, day and time of day.

- **They just forget about the battle so it doesn't matter.**
  Many people who are forced to bathe stay upset for hours.

- **Regulators, advocates and families will see it as possible neglect.**
  When you are rethinking what is currently accepted practice, be proactive and educate all players. Let people know what you are doing and why. Frame it as a better way of meeting someone's needs.

- **The individualized approach will take more time and we don't have it.**
  For most people, if you are organized, have your supplies handy and are familiar with the techniques, it can be done in the same amount of time. If overall, you end up bathing some people less frequently, then there may be a decrease in time spent bathing.

OVERHEAD

Bed Bath

Consider a bed bath for persons who are:

- frail (who fatigue easily);
- nonambulatory;
- experience pain on transfer;
- fearful of lifts;
- experiencing acute illness;
- afraid of the shower spray;
- overstimulated in the shower;
- expressing desire for it.

OVERHEAD

Towel Bath

1. Prepare the person.
2. Prepare the bath.
3. Bathe the person.
4. Allow person to rest.

OVERHEAD

Individualizing the Towel Bath

Concern	Action
• cold	• cover with dry towel • double bag wet towel • remove wet towel quickly
• pain when turning over	• wash back, rectum, and genitals while standing
• agitation	• have one person talk while a second one washes • use other distracters • keep lights low • play soft music

Case Example

Mr. Nash is a 75-year-old man who is severely demented. He is incontinent of bowel and bladder and can speak very few words. He yells every time you try to move him. He cries throughout his shower and is difficult to console. He seems to be sensitive to cold as he keeps trying to cover himself. His daughter visits every day and is concerned about his health and well-being.

Case Example

Mrs. Pearl is a very active woman in the middle stage of Alzheimer's disease. She wanders the halls during the day, greets people with a smile and then moves on. She enjoys dancing and loves "Big Band" music. She is very agitated during the shower. She keeps trying to get up out of the chair and leave the bathroom. Her rectum is very sensitive due to hemorrhoids and she yells and squirms when it is being washed.

CHAPTER 13

Taking Care of Yourself: Strategies for Caregivers

Joyce H. Rasin

THE STRESSES OF CAREGIVING

As a care provider, you spend many hours a day attending to other people. But how much time do you actually spend caring for yourself? Caring for yourself is as important as caring for others. Caregiving can be rewarding and challenging. However, providing care to persons with dementia who have behavioral symptoms can be stressful. Stress occurs when you experience the daily events in your life as potentially harmful (e.g., leading to loss) or when you see the challenges in your life as difficult, painful, or unfair. Stress also occurs when you are concerned that you may not have the resources to cope with these events or the daily "hassles" of caregiving. Stressors in your life can be personal, interpersonal, or environmental. Typical daily stressors for paid care providers include:

- Mr. H. continually begs you not to give him a shower. It makes you feel really bad that you have to continue, but it has to be done because it is his bath day.
- When you try to wash Ms. P's hair she pushes your hand away and calls you a name.
- Mr. M. starts to cry when you tell him he can't go home.
- Ms. R. moans whenever you move her leg.
- Your schedule changes with little notice.
- You have a disagreement with a supervisor or co-worker.
- The shower room is too hot.
- There are not enough towels or washcloths to do the job well.

Typical daily stressors for family care providers include:

- Your husband doesn't recognize you when you come to assist him with bathing.
- Your mother is up all night wandering in the house and you are fearful she will get out and get lost.
- Your wife is no longer safe in the kitchen and you don't know how to cook or use the appliances.
- You have to cut through the red tape of health insurance carriers.
- You are having trouble finding a sitter so you can go to the doctor.

Recognizing those situations you find stressful is the first step in dealing with them. If the stress you experience from caregiving is not minimized or reduced, your physical, emotional, and/or social health may be affected. Once you recognize the source of your stress, you can begin to find ways to manage your reaction to it.

Personal Stress Responses

Sometimes as a care provider, you are so focused on the care receiver that you don't notice your own feelings. Throughout your day you have moments when you feel stressed and others when you feel relaxed. Try to become aware of the first sign of stress so it won't increase. Think about your typical day. To identify some of the ways that you respond to stressors, complete "Personal Reaction to Stress" in Table 13.1.

TABLE 13.1 Personal Reaction to Stress

When you're feeling stressed and anxious, what do you typically experience? Check all that apply.

_____	1. My heart beats faster.
_____	2. I get diarrhea.
_____	3. I have sweaty palms.
_____	4. I lose my appetite.
_____	5. I feel anxious.
_____	6. I become very critical of other people.
_____	7. I tend to cry.
_____	8. I withdraw from my family and friends.
_____	9. I become forgetful.
_____	10. I lose my concentration easily.
_____	11. I can't get as much done as usual.
_____	12. I lose interest.

You can respond to stress with your body (physically), through your feelings (emotionally), or in your thinking (cognitively). All of these responses are normal responses and let you know that you are reacting to something that you, consciously or unconsciously, view as a stressor. In the "Personal Reaction to Stress" checklist, physical responses are #1, 2, 3, and 4; emotional responses are #5, 6, 7, and 8; and cognitive responses are #9, 10, 11, and 12. You may have more responses that are physical, whereas another person will have more emotional responses. It is also possible to have responses from all categories. The type and the number of your responses will differ from other people's responses. Being aware of your reactions can help you develop ways to care for yourself.

Burnout

All caregivers are at risk of burnout. You may be on the verge of burning out when the stressors you experience from caregiving overpower your ability to cope with them. Burnout may result from chronic stressful situations also. The classic symptoms of burnout are loss of energy and enthusiasm, increased dissatisfaction, pessimism, and inefficiency. You may feel overloaded or as if you don't know what you are doing anymore. Burnout increases your risk for developing physical problems such as high blood pressure and heart disease, or emotional problems such as depression. Burnout begins slowly and increases gradually, so catching it early

is important. See Table 13.2 for some warning signs that a stressful situation is overwhelming your ability to cope with it, and that you are burning out.

If one or more of the above signs occurs frequently, you are a candidate for burnout. Turn to a close friend or confidant, or ask your primary health care provider or spiritual advisor for assistance in coping with your stressors. Many people try to relieve their stress by smoking, excessive drinking, overeating, or taking unnecessary pills. These actions also can have a negative impact on your health. Before you begin to experience signs of burnout, you can make a health care plan for yourself. Incorporate into your lifestyle some alternative strategies for coping with stress.

Strategies for Self-Care

Develop a plan for self-care to prevent or diminish stress in your life. Some strategies are appropriate for all care providers whereas others are specific to either paid or family care providers. You may find some of the following strategies helpful for your self-care plan.

Strategies for All Care Providers

Physical Health

Staying physically healthy will help you to stay emotionally healthy. Your health is one of the most im-

TABLE 13.2 Signs of Burnout

How often do these occur?

		Never	Sometimes	Frequently
1.	Coming down with more colds and headaches than usual.	❐	❐	❐
2.	Can't get excited about your job.	❐	❐	❐
3.	Don't enjoy giving care to care receiver.	❐	❐	❐
4.	Lie awake at night worrying.	❐	❐	❐
5.	Suddenly losing weight without trying.	❐	❐	❐
6.	Frequent conflicts with care receiver, coworkers, and/or family.	❐	❐	❐
7.	Crying every day.	❐	❐	❐
8.	Resent suggestions from coworkers and family for doing things.	❐	❐	❐
9.	Feeling tired all day.	❐	❐	❐

portant resources that you have and is essential if you want to be a long-term care provider. So there are two reasons to maintain your health—for your own well-being and for the well-being of the person(s) for whom you care. Diet, exercise, and sleep will improve your ability to cope with the stress you experience from caregiving.

A balanced diet is important for good health. Every day you should have:

- grains;
- fruits and vegetables;
- milk, cheese, or yogurt;
- poultry, fish, meat, eggs, or dried beans;
- 2 quarts of water;
- sugar in moderation;
- no more than one alcoholic drink;
- low fat and cholesterol.

Choose foods in each category that you like. Take time to relax as you eat. Try not to read or watch television while eating so you can be aware of the flavors. Food is a necessity and a pleasure, so enjoy!

Regular exercise. Pick an activity that you enjoy. Three types of exercises are important for physical fitness:

- Endurance or aerobic.
- Strengthening or muscle building.
- Flexibility.

Endurance/aerobic exercises increase your heart and lung function and should be done at least three times per week. Walking, swimming, biking, and dancing are all aerobic exercises. Start slowly and increase the intensity gradually. Even a five-minute walk a day is a good start. If you can't talk while you are exercising, you are going too fast. See your physician or other primary health care provider before you begin your routine if you have heart trouble, chest pain, diabetes, high blood pressure, dizziness, or arthritis. To complete your fitness program include exercises to strengthen your muscles (lifting weights such as hand weights, soup cans, or water bottles) and to stretch your muscles. The National Institute on Aging puts out an excellent exercise guide that is available for free and a videotape for a small fee (see resources at the end of this chapter). Many video stores and libraries also have exercise videos.

Sleep. Getting an adequate number of hours of sleep is very important. Many people in the United States are sleep deprived and fail to get 8 hours of sleep a night (National Sleep Foundation, 1998). Sleep is a time for your mind and your body to rest. Having good sleep habits (regular bedtime and comfortable room environment) will help you to rest. Try not to read or watch television in bed so that going to bed is associated with going to sleep.

Learning to Relax

Learning to physically and mentally relax is an important skill to develop. Two ways to relax are "attending to simple pleasures" and "achieving the relaxation response."

Attend to the simple pleasures in your life. Simple pleasures are activities that bring a smile to your face and a feeling of contentment. They are not expensive, nor do they take time to plan. They allow you to appreciate what is happening to you in the moment and not worry about the past or the future. Some examples of simple pleasures are:

- Walking through a wooded area in the fall where all you can hear is the crunching of leaves from the pressure of your footsteps.
- Filling the tub full of warm water, adding favorite bubble bath or bath oil, soft music in the background, a burning candle, and a pillow for your neck and head. (Spend about 20 minutes of solitude in your bath.)
- Sharing a funny story with a friend.

Identify some simple pleasures for yourself and build them into your daily routine. Enjoy them throughout the day.

Caregiver Wisdom

It's important to focus on the person but if I'm distracted by worries, I stop for a minute, talk to myself, and then refocus.
Rosa Stephens, CNA, Oxford Manor, Oxford, NC

The relaxation response is a physical state of rest that alters the physical and emotional response to stress.

TABLE 13.3   The Relaxation Response

- Select your focus word(s)—a word with special meaning for you.
- Sit quietly in a comfortable position.
- Close your eyes.
- Let your muscles go limp, stretch to let go of any tension.
- Breathe slowly and naturally. Repeat your focus words as you exhale.
- When other thoughts come into your head, just ignore them and return to your focus word(s).
- Continue for 10-20 minutes each time.
- When you are finished, don't stand immediately but sit quietly for a minute and let your everyday thoughts return.

Since the early 1960s, Dr. Herbert Benson and colleagues (2000) have been teaching persons how to elicit this response as part of a program to decrease stress-related medical disorders. If the body can relax, the mind will follow. Just two things must be completed: 1) selecting a focus word, phrase, or prayer such as "Peace," "Calm," "Relax," "Om," "The Lord is my shepherd"; and 2) disregarding everyday thoughts that come to mind. See Table 13.3 for steps to achieve the relaxation response.

Support Network

Throughout this book the importance of the caregiving relationship has been emphasized. Supportive relationships help to minimize the effects of all types of stressors, including those associated with providing care. Find a person or persons whom you can confide in or with whom you feel comfortable talking. Confidants can be found among your coworkers, family members, or friends. These individuals can not only provide emotional support, they can also help you learn new problem solving skills.

Attitudes and Beliefs

Positive self-talks. Your thoughts influence your feelings. In other words, what you tell yourself is what you will feel. If you are involved in negative self-talk, you are encouraging yourself to feel negative. To prepare for using positive self-talk, write down some positive statements about yourself. For example, "I did a really good job getting Mr. M. to change his clothes." "I am capable of giving excellent care." When you are feeling

anxious and not good about yourself, take out your statements and read them.

Caregiver Wisdom

I try to keep a positive outlook. I make a list of all the good memories and when I get down, I read that list to remind me of the good things. I depend a lot on my church and spiritual beliefs to give me support. I attend Bible study classes. I garden. Those are all therapeutic for me.

Pat Ehresman, in-home caregiver for her mother, who has Parkinson's disease, and her husband, who has dementia

Professional Counseling and Therapy

If you have tried everything suggested here and still feel physically or emotionally exhausted, you may benefit from professional assistance to help you identify positive steps to manage your stress. Some people you could contact if you decide you need help include:

- Priest, pastor, or rabbi.
- Your physician or primary care provider.
- Clinical psychologist, psychiatric mental health nurses specialist, or social worker. Many of these health professionals can be found at a local mental health clinic.

Strategies Specifically for Paid Care Providers

As paid care providers, your situation is a little different from that of family care providers. The long-term care of several persons who may have mental and/or physical impairments can be very stressful. Adding a stressful work situation to everyday life may make coping more difficult. Consider the following in addition to the strategies already discussed in this chapter.

- *Support at work*
  Support at work can be informal or organized. Talking with a coworker from another unit or floor, who isn't involved in your immediate caregiving situation, can provide you with a nonjudgmental listener. By talking through the situation,

you may view it in a different way. Support can be supplied more formally through team meetings, team venting sessions, or your clinical supervisor in a positive work environment. Having colleagues who not only listen to your frustrations but also provide feedback and help with problem solving can be very beneficial.

- *Change.* You may have talked with coworkers and clinical managers/supervisors about a difficult situation with a care receiver. You may have brainstormed about different ways to resolve the situation and tried alternative approaches. However, sometimes because of other stressors occurring in your life, you are not as resilient and may need some respite. Talk with your clinical supervisor about a short-term change in assignment.

- *Relax.* Yes, it is possible to relax at work. On your break, if the weather allows, go outside for a few minutes and enjoy the sun, the wind, or even the rain. Forget about what else you have to do and be aware of your surroundings. Give your body and your mind a chance to slow down. Pause, breathe deeply a few times, smile, and let your body relax.

Caregiver Wisdom

When stressed at work, we would talk among ourselves and try to work it out. We tried to support each other. I also found the nurses and doctors helpful. I could talk to them about personal or work-related issues.

Tom Pruitt, HCT, retired from John Umstead Hospital, Butner, NC

Strategies Specifically for Family Care Providers

- *Be realistic about what is possible.* There is a limit to what any one person can do within one day. First, you have to differentiate between needs and wants. Although you may have a list of things you want done, all of them may not need to be done. Needs and wants will differ by family and

only you can make the choice. What you value most is what is important, not what others think. Even after you identify your needs, you still may have to set limits on what you can do within a day. Be realistic and don't be afraid to ask for assistance.

Caregiver Wisdom

I accept my new limitations. I recognize that I don't have the same level of freedom that I had before. I can't just go off shopping or visiting with friends. I have to plan ahead for those things to happen now and it is helpful that I have come to accept that this is true and that I have to ask for help to get away when I need to. I have also come to accept the new limitations of my mother and husband. I have dropped all expectations about how they were or should be and recognize that they have changed and I need to adjust. It makes life easier.

Pat Ehresman, in-home caregiver for her mother, who has Parkinson's disease, and her husband, who has dementia

---

- *Get help from your family and friends.* How often has someone told you to "Let me know when I can help you"? Many times other people want to help, but they don't know how they can be of assistance. They need some direction. Make a list of what needs to be done. Perhaps you need someone to sit with your family member while you do errands or so that you can focus on an activity within your home without an interruption. Make sure some of the activities on the list are for your self-care. Taking a walk, going to the movies, or taking a nap. Asking for help is actually strength, not a weakness. You can't do it alone.

- *Share your feelings with others.* Being able to share feelings with a close friend or family member helps to get them out in the open and to lessen the impact of negative emotions. Pick someone with whom you can confide or comfortably talk without censoring your feelings. Many care providers also have gained strength through support by different organizations such as the Alzheimer' Association, American Heart Association, and

American Cancer Society. Check the newspaper for listings of meetings. Care providers who belong to a faith community may find that the spiritual leader (priest, pastor, rabbi) can provide guidance.

Gender Differences

Traditionally, most family caregivers have been women. However, as the population ages and people live longer, more men are finding themselves in caregiving roles by choice or circumstance. Men may have some different issues. They have lost their key source of emotional support if the care receiver is their spouse. In addition, because traditionally they have not been responsible for the day-to-day homemaking chores, they may be at a loss. Men may benefit from a support group for men only and community resources for meals, personal care, housecleaning, and shopping. The local Area Agency for Aging provides information and referral services. See "Eldercare Locator" on the resource list.

SUMMARY

Being a sensitive care provider has the potential to be stressful. If you find that you are experiencing stress from the caregiving, develop a plan for self-care. Without a plan for self-care, you may become overwhelmed or burned out which could result in physical and emotional problems. Several strategies have been described that can either decrease your vulnerability to stress or help you manage and cope with stressful situations. Evaluate your use of self-care strategies by answering the questions in Table 13.4. Then, list three strategies below that you can include in your plan for self-care.

Strategies Selected for My Self-Care

1. _____
2. _____
3. _____

See resources at the end of this chapter for sources of additional information. Remember, you need to take care of yourself if you are going to care for others over the long haul. Finding meaning and pleasure in caregiving will be your reward.

TABLE 13.4 Self-Care Strategies

Directions: Read each statement. How often do they occur now?

	Never	Sometimes	Frequently
1. I eat at least one hot, balanced meal a day.	❑	❑	❑
2. I get seven to eight hours sleep a night.	❑	❑	❑
3. I give and receive affection regularly.	❑	❑	❑
4. I exercise at least three times a week.	❑	❑	❑
5. I take fewer than five alcoholic drinks a week.	❑	❑	❑
6. I am the appropriate weight for my height.	❑	❑	❑
7. I get strength from my spiritual beliefs.	❑	❑	❑
8. I am regularly involved in a social activity.	❑	❑	❑
9. I have a network of friends and acquaintances.	❑	❑	❑
10. I have one or more friends to confide in about personal matters.	❑	❑	❑
11. I am able to speak openly about my feelings when angry or worried.	❑	❑	❑
12. I do something for fun on a regular basis.	❑	❑	❑
13. I am able to organize my time effectively.	❑	❑	❑
14. I take quiet time for myself during the day.	❑	❑	❑

TOTAL

Count the number of "Frequently" responses. How many do you have? _____

What can you do to change "Never" to "Frequently"?

Choose three strategies to use as part of your self-care plan.

REFERENCES

Benson, H. (2000, March 18). *Testimony of Herbert Benson M.D. regarding the establishment of HCFA Demonstration Projects to test the efficacy of mind-body medicine before the United States Senate Appropriations Subcommittee* [On-line]. Available: www.senate.gov/~appropriations/labor/testimony/benson.htm.

National Sleep Foundation. *1998 Survey of American women.* [On-line]. Available: http://ww.med.stanford.edu/school/psychiatry/coe/, 1/01.

Seward, B. L. (1999). *Stressed is desserts spelled backward.* Berkeley: Conari Press.

Sime, W. E. (2000, October 19). *Stress management. A review of the principles.* [On-line]. Available: http://libind.unl.edu/stress/mgmt.

APPENDIX

Resources

Several website locations are provided. As long as you use sites developed by reputable organizations and agencies, they are a good source of current, reliable and free information. If you don't have access to the Internet, many local public libraries have it available. Ask your librarian to help you locate the Web page.

Administration on Aging—Has an online resource guide for care providers called "Because We Care," www.aoa.dhhs.gov/wecare.

Alzheimer's Association
70 E. Lake Street, Suite 600
Chicago, IL 60601
1-800-621-0379
http://www.alz.org

Alzheimer's Disease Education and Referral Center
An information specialist can help you obtain information about dementia and related services.
1-800-438-4380

American Association for Retired Persons
On their website, under the category of life transitions, there is a section called "Caregiving." One of the articles in this section is about managing stress.
www.aarp.org

American Heart Association (information about strokes)
7320 Greenville Ave.
Dallas, TX 75231
Local chapters have information for family care providers.
www.americanheart.org
They also have an online "Fitness Center" that includes information about evaluating fitness and an exercise diary.
www.justmove.org

County or city:
Social services department
Mental health department
(Check telephone book for local listings.)

Eldercare Locator
Can direct at no charge to the nearest Area Agency on Aging that knows local resources for housekeeping, personal care services, Meals on Wheels.
1-800-677-1116
www.aoa.gov/elderpage/locator.html

Food and Nutrition Information Center of the U.S. Department of Agriculture
Food Guide Pyramid Booklet updated 2000.
www.nal.usda.gov/fnic

Mayo Clinic: Caring for the Care Provider: Tips on Reducing Stress
www.mayo.edu/geriatrics-rst

National Alliance for Caregiving
4720 Montgomery Lane Suite 642
Bethesda, MD 20814
http://www.caregiving.org

National Institute on Aging
Has exercise video and 100-page companion book for $7.
1-800-222-2225
http://www.nih.gov/nia/health

National Institute for Occupational Safety and Health
Provides information and publications about job stress.
1-800-356-4674
http://www.cdc.gov/niosh/jobstress.html

National Family Care Providers Association
10605 Concord Street, Suite 501
Kensington, MD 20895-2504
1-800-896-3650
http://www.nfcares.org

National Mental Health Association
Can refer to a local specialist.
1-800-969-6642
http://www.nmha.org

Pillemer, K. *The Nursing Assistant's Survival Guide.* For a description see the publishers website: http:www.frontlinepub.com or call 1-800-348-0605.

Measuring Success: A Quality Improvement Program for Individualized Bathing

Anytime you are trying to change practice, it is useful and necessary to determine a practical, valid, and reliable way to measure effectiveness. A formal complex study is not necessary, but some way of monitoring success is. Here are some suggested ways that this could be done with bathing as a Quality Improvement Program. In this model, each person acts as his or her own control and data is collected before and after an intervention. A direct caregiver working with a supervisor or educator will do most of the work. This two-person team will meet regularly, review progress, generate new ideas, and test them out. A program like this addresses OBRA-87 guidelines for nursing home settings and is often favorably received by state surveyors. Plus your staff will improve in their ability to solve care problems.

FOCUS ON THE PERSON BEING BATHED

1. **Select the person(s) for whom you wish to create an individualized bathing approach.**

   As mentioned in chapter 11, it may be useful to start with one or two people in one section of the facility and expand later. It is also helpful to start with less complicated behaviors and persons. Choose a person with strengths you can use such as the ability to understand what you say. Don't pick your most challenging resident. Wait until you have gained some experience.

2. **Select the caregiver(s) who will be working with each person being bathed.**

   Select one caregiver to work with each person being bathed. If two or more caregivers are needed, it is helpful to have a consistent second person. This is not crucial as long as the primary person is the same and guides the interaction. This primary person should be someone who is interested in learning new methods for making bathing pleasurable.

3. **Decide what target behaviors you wish to alter for each person and set measurable goals.**

   These can be positive behaviors you wish to increase or negative behaviors you wish to decrease (Table 4.1). You are identifying how you will know if your approaches are successful; in other words, what you want to change.

4. **Decide on an observational method to measure change.**

   Here are some suggested ways to measure change in the behaviors of the person being bathed:

   a. Direct observation: Have an uninvolved staff person present when the person is being bathed. Choose this person carefully, as he or she will need to be objective and unbiased. Develop a form that lists your target behaviors and ask the person to count them during the bath. The Behavior Checklist (Appendix B) could be used for this.

b. Recalling and recording: Ask the bathing caregiver(s) to recall target behaviors and record them on a form. The Behavior Checklist (Appendix B) could be used for this.

c. Videotaping: As mentioned earlier, videotaping the bath can be a useful learning tool. It can also be used as a method of measuring outcomes. Obtain written permission from the family and verbal assent from the person before each bath. Tape three baseline (pretest) and three postintervention (posttest baths). Then ask a staff member (who is actively involved in the resident's care) to view the tapes without knowledge of which tape was pre and which was post. This is a stronger methodology for evaluation as it eliminates some potential bias. The Behavior Checklist could be used to count resident behaviors. Great caution must be used to insure the confidentiality of the tapes and who views them. They must be destroyed when the evaluation is complete.

Each method has pros and cons. The direct observation requires an extra person. The recall method relies on the memory of an involved and, therefore, potentially biased participant. The videotaping may be seen as too intrusive and time-consuming.

5. Decide on any physiologic measures you wish to monitor.

Identify the physical concerns (odor, overall appearance, skin problems, etc) you have related to changing the bathing program for the person. Develop a data collection method. These may be very simple such as a narrative note or a scale from 0-3. If you use a scale, having descriptors and definitions for each point on the scale will make it easier to use. For example, 0 could be labeled as "0" or "no odor", and 3 could be labeled as "a lot" or "very strong odor." These labels "anchor" the points on the scale and helps clarify what each one means.

6. Collect your baseline data.

Baseline data is information collected before you try a new method or approach. Have the caregiver(s) bathe the person in the usual way (tub, shower, bed bath). Collect data using your chosen method for 3 baths.

7. Decide on possible causes/triggers for behaviors.

Following the collection of the baseline data, you will need to provide some education and training (see chapter 12) for the intervention team (the direct caregiver and the supervisor or educator.) They will then brainstorm and problem solve **before the next bath.** You may find the Behavior Tracking Log (Figure 3.1) and Bathing Preferences and Practices Form (Appendix, chapter 3) helpful. The baseline data will also be helpful for you to use in problem solving.

8. Select solutions/approaches you wish to try.

Chapter 4 will be very useful in helping you decide on new interventions for the specific problems you have identified. Check the tables that are available for problems such as pain, being cold, refusing to enter bathing room for solutions. Use the Intervention Planning Table (Appendix, chapter 4) as a tool.

9. Test solutions.

With the next bath, the designated caregiver will try out the selected solutions. Following each bath or shower, those involved will debrief and brainstorm and evaluate the selected interventions. Again, the Intervention Planning Table (Appendix, chapter 4) will be useful. Decide what worked, what didn't work and why and what you will try next time.

10. Finalize your care plan.

Continue this process for several baths or until the caregiver feels that he/she has reached the goals set for the target behaviors, or has run out of ideas/solutions. The number of trials needed to finalize the care plan will vary from person to person. The average is about 3-4 times but some person's discomfort can be reduced in one time. For others, some discomfort and distress may remain. Six to eight attempts to revise care approaches are probably a sufficient trial. Write up an individualized bathing care plan that the caregiver will follow during the posttest data collection period.

11. Collect your postintervention or posttest data.

Using the same data collection method you used for the baseline baths, collect data on the next 3 baths, with the caregiver(s) using the individualized bathing care plan developed in the intervention/solution testing process.

12. Analyze your data.

Look at the data you collected before the intervention and after the intervention was introduced, comparing the counts on the targeted behaviors between the two time periods. Average the scores or numbers for the behaviors observed in the baseline baths and do the same for the behaviors observed in the baths completed after the intervention was introduced. Compare the pretest scores with the posttest scores. Was there an overall increase in positive behaviors and decrease in negative behaviors? If so, the intervention was helpful. If not, it was not successful. Use the data and the insights of the team to decide what the next step should be.

13. Share the results with other involved parties.

Use the data to further your goal of creating a positive bathing experience for all residents and staff. Chart the results to show the outcomes. If you are in a nursing home setting, you may wish to share the study with state surveyors. Also, include this information in the resident's medical chart so that other caregivers will be aware of what worked and what didn't work and progress that has been made toward goals.

FOCUS ON CAREGIVER BEHAVIORS

So far the focus on analysis and study has been on the person being bathed. As we have stated in the book, that is only half of the equation. The actions of the caregiver and the quality of the relationship are a major factor in determining the outcome. The same intervention carried out by caregivers with different styles and motivations can yield very different results.

If you wish to also evaluate the caregiver's behavior, use the direct observation or the videotape method. Using the same approach as described for the person being bathed, ask the observer to fill out the Caregiver Behavior Checklist (Appendix C) for baseline (pretest) and postintervention (posttest) baths. An unbiased observer is very important here also. For the videotaped method, the rater would watch the video a second time to rate the caregiver using the checklist. The observer may also wish to compare the observed caregiver's actions against the written care plan and make an estimate of the percent of the care plan carried out during the bath. This method of data collection will help you gather databased evidence to guide you in implementing and evaluating a care plan.

Behavior Rating Checklist

Name: _____ Date: _____ Time: _____ Recorder: _____

Record the frequency of each behavior by placing an x in the box beside the behavior each time it occurs. If two behaviors occur simultaneously, rate BOTH. Definitions are on the next page.

Behaviors suggesting discomfort*

Frequency	Behavior
	Avoid bathing
	Biting
	Closed fist
	Complaints
	Finger-pointing
	Grabbing or attempts to grab
	Hitting, pushing, scratching, punching, or attempts
	Hostile language
	Kicks or attempts to kick
	Leaving
	Spitting
	Throwing things
	Other agitated or aggressive behavior

Behaviors indicating comfort

Frequency	Behavior
	Hugging/kissing
	Smiling/laughing
	Singing
	Thanks or compliments caregiver
	Other positive behaviors (list)

*HIGHLIGHT BEHAVIORS THAT OCCURRED DURING THE BASELINE BATHS. DID THESE BEHAVIORS IMPROVE?

OVERALL ASSESSMENT OF PERSON'S DISCOMFORT

1	2	3	4	5	6

Completely comfortable   Extremely uncomfortable

Comments: (note anything unusual or surprising that occurred) _____

_____

DEFINITIONS OF BEHAVIORS

Avoiding bathing	resists being bathe, e.g., moves body to avoid being bathed, turns head away when face is being washed, includes avoiding being undressed. If the resident grabs the caregiver, rate as grabbing.
Biting	bites, or attempts to bite, chomps, gnaws (on caregiver only)
Closed fist	closes one or both fists
Complaints	expresses displeasure in words (e.g., "I am cold")
Finger-pointing	points finger at caregiver
Grabbing	grabs or attempts to grab onto people or objects inappropriately; snatches, seizes roughly. DO NOT rate if resident is already grabbing object/person unless resident grabs object/person with other hand. Do not rate if resident is holding on for safety reasons.
Hitting, pushing, scratching	physically abuses or attempts to abuse caregiver with hand or handheld object or with other body parts (head, whole body), includes pushing, shoving, scratching (contact occurs)
Hostile language	cursing/obscene/vulgar language, verbal threats, name-calling
Hugging/Kissing	resident hugs or kisses caregiver
Kicking or attempts to kick	strikes forcefully with foot or leg (contact occurs) or swings out leg and foot with force towards caregiver
Leaving	tries to get out of shower area or resists going to shower area. This is "escape" behavior. REQUIRES caregiver intervention, the caregiver may block an exit with his/her body, may take hold of the resident to keep them in the shower, may pull/push on the resident to get them to walk to the shower.
Sings	sings or hums
Spitting	spits on purpose (does not have to be at caregiver)
Other agitation or aggression	shows physical signs of distress including repetitive mannerisms, hyperactivity, wringing hands, flailing arms, nonpurposeful movement of the feet, legs or torso
Thanks or compliments caregiver	expresses appreciation to caregiver; expresses praise and/or admiration
Throwing things	forcefully throws object, knocks object off surface

Caregiver Behavior Checklist

Name of caregiver: _____ Person being bathed: _____ Date of bath: _____

	Never	Almost Never	Occasionally	Often	Almost Always	Always
VERBAL COMMUNICATION						
Praises resident	1	2	3	4	5	6
Uses a calm voice	1	2	3	4	5	6
Speaks respectfully	1	2	3	4	5	6
Expresses Concern/interest	1	2	3	4	5	6
Speaks directly to resident	1	2	3	4	5	6
TASK PRESENTATION						
Prepares resident for the task	1	2	3	4	5	6
Bathes at a pace appropriate for this resident	1	2	3	4	5	6
NONVERBAL COMMUNICATION						
Gently touches resident	1	2	3	4	5	6
Is flexible with the bathing routine	1	2	3	4	5	6
Makes eye contact with the resident	1	2	3	4	5	6
INDEPENDENCE (assess if appropriate)						
Encourages independence	1	2	3	4	5	6

TOTAL: _____

CAREGIVER BEHAVIOR CHECKLIST DEFINITIONS

RATING SCALE

NEVER: The behavior never occurs.
ALMOST NEVER: The behavior occurs a few times during the bath.
OCCASIONALLY: The behavior occurs less than half of the time.
OFTEN: The behavior occurs more than half the time, OR all of the time through the first half of the bath and never during the second half of the bath.
ALMOST ALWAYS: The behavior occurs all but a few times.
ALWAYS: The behavior occurs all of the time during the whole bath.

VERBAL COMMUNICATION

Praises Resident: The caregiver recognizes the resident's progress, achievement, or cooperation at any time during the bath including prior to undressing. Various forms of praise may include direct reinforcement ("Good job!"), encouragement ("That's right"), or compliments ("You smell nice"). Also used when the caregiver encourages the resident ("You can do it!").

Uses a Calm Voice: A calm voice is slow, smooth, soothing, and the words flow, although it is not necessarily soft, and may be lower in pitch than the caregiver's usual tone. A tense voice is agitated, angry, short and strained. It is possible to speak loudly (so that the resident can hear) and calmly.

Speaks Respectfully: Respectful statements and/or tone of voice imply a position of equality between the resident and caregiver, and relay a sense to the resident that he/she is valued and well thought of. The resident is not made to feel inferior to the caregiver. The resident is spoken to in a disrespectful manner when the caregiver is unnecessarily authoritative, impolite, or discourteous. This includes the use of commands (i.e., "Sit down!" vs. "Please take a seat.") A disrespectful speaking manner endangers the resident's self-worth and dignity. Examples of disrespectful manner include "talking down" to the resident as if he or she was a child, making derogatory comments to/about the resident, and "making fun" of or mocking the resident. Sugary, sweet speech should not be rated as disrespectful.

Expresses Concern/Interest: This item is rated as expressing concern/interest regarding the bathing tasks only. An interested caregiver is concerned with the resident's immediate well-being and shows a genuine caring attitude toward the resident's immediate feelings and condition as related to the bath. For example, the caregiver may ask the resident about his or her comfort, the temperature of the water, if the resident is cold, etc. A caregiver who is uninterested does not ask about how the resident is feeling and never addresses these issues in a verbal manner.

Speaks Directly to Resident: Response choices on this item indicate how much the caregiver talks to the resident regardless of the topic (i.e., giving bathing instructions, conversation as a means of distraction, etc.). All other conversation not related to the bathing task (i.e., asking about the resident's family, discussing the weather, holidays, etc.) is rated under this item. This item addresses how much the caregiver speaks to the resident overall.

TASK PRESENTATION STYLE

Prepares Resident for the Task: Caregiver tells the resident about the next task that he or she is about to perform before it is initiated (i.e., putting water on resident, washing the face, placing a washcloth over the resident's eyes and stating that she will rinse the hair). This does not include incidents when the caregiver is requesting that the resident perform a task (e.g., "Wash your face"). Note this item is rated in proportion to the amount of times the caregiver assists the resident. If the resident is mostly independent in bathing, but the caregiver assists with one task and prepares the resident for this task, this category is rated always.

Bathes at a Pace Appropriate for This Resident. The caregiver adjusts the pace of the bath to meet the needs of the resident. This means speeding up if the resident asks the caregiver to do so or slowing down to give the resident time to understand requests. A bath that is too hurried is characterized by the rapid introduction and implementation of each step in the bathing process. An example of a hurried bath is when two caregivers are present and they are simultaneously washing the resident. This bathing style may also minimize the resident's participation. An unhurried bath progresses slowly with, perhaps, some resident involvement.

NONVERBAL COMMUNICATION

Gently Touches Resident: A gentle touch is light, physical contact with the resident during all assistance. An example of intermediate touch is firm, sustained contact (e.g., holding resident's arm) used in order to guide resident. Rough touch is abrasive and involves unnecessary, hard pressure (e.g., forcefully holding resident down, roughly removing clothes). Rough touch may also be relatively speedy and vigorous (e.g., "scrubbing" resident).

Is Flexible with the Bathing Routine: A caregiver who exhibits flexibility is willing to change his or her bathing routine in order to accommodate the resident's needs especially, but not only, during incidents of resident verbal uncooperativeness (e.g., complaints) and/or physical uncooperativeness (e.g., hitting, refusing to sit in the tub). A flexible caregiver is willing to "work around" the resident, delay tasks, and try new strategies in order to gain compliance. Physical manipulation after several attempts to gain compliance with one strategy should not be considered inflexible. An inflexible caregiver is unwilling to change his or her bathing routine in order to meet the needs of the resident. Inflexibility may involve forcing the resident to comply, and/or unnecessarily manipulating the resident into potentially awkward and uncomfortable positions in order to accommodate the caregiver's routine (e.g., forcing the resident to walk across the room to sit in a chair instead of bringing the chair to the resident). In order to rate this item, the resident must indicate that she/he needs a change. This indication may be verbal (asking for a change, saying no, screaming, yelling) or physical (pushing away, hitting, kicking, asserting independence). Caregivers who allow residents to go back and wash body parts that have already been washed are rated as exhibiting flexibility.

Makes Eye Contact with the Resident: This includes attempts to make eye contact even when the resident is unresponsive to the attempts. This item requires that the resident and caregiver are facing each other.

INDEPENDENCE:

Encourages Independence: Caregiver attempts to encourage and/or allow the resident to perform or assist in bathing tasks. For example, the caregiver places a washcloth in the resident's hand and asks her to wash her face, arms, legs, etc. This item is not appropriate if the resident is unable to move or assist in any way.

Index